Communication in Health Care

A skills-based approach

Henry A. Minardi
BSc (Hons) Psychology, Diploma in Counselling and Supervision, Diploma in Nursing, Cert Ed, RGN, RMN
Senior Lecturer, Faculty of Health Studies, Middlesex University; previously Practice Development Tutor, Bethlem and Maudsley NHS Trust, UK

Martin J. Riley
MA Counselling Studies, BA (Hons) Health Studies, Cert Ed, RGN, RMN
Counsellor Co-ordinator, Psychology Department, Clwydian Community Care Trust, North Wales, UK

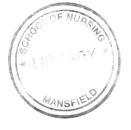
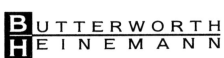
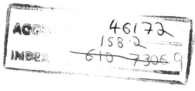

BUTTERWORTH
HEINEMANN

Butterworth-Heinemann
Linacre House, Jordan Hill, Oxford OX2 8DP
A division of Reed Educational and Professional Publishing Ltd

A member of the Reed Elsevier plc group

OXFORD   BOSTON   JOHANNESBURG
MELBOURNE   NEW DELHI   SINGAPORE

First published 1997

© Reed Educational and Professional Publishing Ltd 1997

British Library Cataloguing in Publication Data
A catalogue record for this book is available from the British Library

Library of Congress Cataloguing in Publication Data
A catalogue record for this book is available from the Library of Congress

ISBN 0 7506 1579 6

Typeset by Latimer Trend & Co Ltd, Plymouth
Printed and bound in Great Britain by Biddles Ltd, Guildford and
King's Lynn

Contents

Acknowledgements

This book evolved from a communications curriculum that was initially developed for student psychiatric nurses. The workshops, and the exercises within them, have been tested and refined over a long period. The feedback from colleagues and students has always been invaluable in helping us to improve the work we were doing and in encouraging us to write this book.

However, the book would not have been possible without the patient perseverance and encouragement of Susan Devlin, the Senior Medical Editor at Butterworth Heinemann. Above all, we would like to thank our families, Jane and Nicholas Minardi, and Gill, Jennifer and Dorcas Riley, for their help, encouragement and tolerance throughout the writing of the book. Particular thanks must go to Jane for examining each of the chapters and offering the 'fine tuning' needed to make the book accessible to a wide readership.

PART I:

Theoretical Overview

Chapter 1

Introduction

'Then you should say what you mean,' the March Hare went on.

'I do,' Alice hastily replied; 'at least – at least I mean what I say – that's the same thing you know.'

'Not the same thing a bit!' said the Hatter. 'You might just as well say that, "I see what I eat" is the same thing as "I eat what I see"!'

'You might just as well say,' added the March Hare, 'that "I like what I get" is the same thing as "I get what I like".'

Alice's Adventures in Wonderland (Lewis Carroll, 1946: p. 94).

Effective health care is about providing for the explicit and implicit health needs of people. This requires that health care workers at all levels should perceive and understand both overt and hidden messages from clients, and receive and transmit communications competently. Unlike Alice, they must be able to recognize the distinction between 'saying what they mean' and 'meaning what they say' as well as understand the meanings of the communications of clients/patients. However, it would be unwise to assume that health care workers will automatically be adept at all appropriate forms of communication in the various situations they are likely to experience. It was in the light of this that we developed a communication skills course containing experiential workshops to prepare students in mental health care settings for work with clients.

This book evolved out of that course. At the heart of it are the skills workshops that we developed over a number of years. It has been written in the belief that all health care workers should have the opportunity to enhance their communication skills and thus be able to 'say what they mean' and 'mean what they say' to patients, thus resulting in more effective health care. At the outset we had not considered writing this book, and were simply concerned with ensuring that students were well prepared. However, over the years – and after continuous positive evaluation from the participants – we concluded that such an active and well received curriculum might be of use to others who are teaching, and learning, within the field of communications.

The delivery of health care has changed radically in recent years; it is now provided in a wide variety of settings and by a broad cross-section of people. Although the material presented in this book was originally designed for nurses, we have broadened the scope of these workshops to reflect the fact that health care is not provided only in traditional settings such as hospitals and clinics, by people in professions such as medicine, nursing, occupational therapy, social work, physiotherapy and clinical psychology. It is now delivered more frequently in social care settings such as day centres, residential facilities and client's homes, by generic care workers and people in the voluntary sector services, as well as by families and friends, who provide physical and emotional support to those in need. To reflect this diversity of provision, we have chosen to use the term 'health care worker' throughout the book so that the focus is not upon any one professional group; we have also attempted to use a broad range of examples. Similarly, we faced the dilemma of choosing a term to describe the recipients of health care, settling eventually upon the term 'client', again to reflect the wide range of settings in which individuals receive health care and to avoid the implied passivity of the term 'patient'.

Health Care Settings and Effective Communication

The World Health Organization's definition of health as physical, mental and social well-being and not just as the absence of illness or infirmity (Nutbeam, 1986) does not help very much in enabling health care workers to clarify the aim of their communication with clients. However, in the UK, recent government conceptualizations of health focus on individual responsibilities, suggesting health consists of

> ... **adding years to life:** an increase in life expectancy and reduction in premature death; and **adding life to years:** increasing years lived free from ill-health, reducing or minimising the adverse effects of illness and disability, promoting healthy lifestyles, physical and social environments and, overall, improving quality of life (Department of Health, 1992: p. 13).

This concept of enhancing quality of life provides a purpose for communication within health care settings and implicitly acknowledges that the concept of health encompasses the belief systems and social values of individuals and their cultures.

Health care settings are often thought of by professionals and nonprofessionals as being synonymous with institutions and health care as the preserve of professionals. However, the changes in health care settings alluded to above have had a number of far-reaching consequences, with the development of broad-based definitions. The National Council for Vocational Qualifications recognizes the wider perspective of health care settings in its definition: 'Care setting: the environment in which care takes place' (Care Sector Consortium, 1992: p. xiii). Thus, a health care worker helping elderly clients to dress in their own homes requires as much skilled communication to get his or her message across as a general practitioner treating patients in the surgery.

Whatever terms are used, our belief is that anyone who takes on the task of caring for someone's health needs requires the opportunity to become a more proficient communicator, thereby enhancing the best resource that they can provide for the client (i.e. themselves).

Theoretical and Educational Aspects of Skilled Communication

This book is presented in two sections. Part I (Chapters 1–4) examines some theoretical issues of communication and the learning of related skills, while Part II (Chapters 5–12) offers an integrated series of communication skills workshops to help practitioners/ carers to improve interactions with their particular client groups.

Part I: Theoretical Overview

In this chapter (Chapter 1) we offer the reader a 'map' of the book as a whole, including an overview of all other chapters. This will enable the reader to select those sections of the book that are most appropriate to individual needs, be it the theoretical issues involved in communication and its teaching, or the skills-based workshops. This chapter additionally provides guidance on the overall structure of the workshops, with recommendations about setting up and facilitating them. We do not suggest that the book should be read from cover to cover – although this may be appropriate for some people – but that readers should choose those sections that meet the developmental, practical and professional needs of themselves and the individuals with whom they work.

In order to understand and use communication skills competently, it is necessary to have a knowledge base (Jarvis, 1988; Minton, 1991; Quinn, 1995); this we provide in Chapter 2, which examines pathways of communication, transmission and reception routes, and the role of personal and environmental factors. This chapter also looks at the constructs of communication (e.g. verbal/nonverbal, linguistic/nonlinguistic, visual/auditory; see Ellis and Beattie, 1986; Sutherland, 1992) and the need for accuracy of communication to meet specific outcomes. In particular we focus upon the components of verbal and nonverbal communication, using the concept of active listening as a bridge connecting these two forms of communication (see Figure 2.3), especially in the field of health care.

The destabilizing effect of ill health can result in an individual responding to previously trivial problems with uncertainty and trepidation. A potential exists for this to increase the individual's difficulties, unless they have identified ways of coping with the stress caused by ill health. Studies have demonstrated that learning coping techniques can improve immunological resistance (see e.g. Arnetz *et al.* 1987; Kiecolt-Glaser *et al.* 1986). Chapter 3 explores the way in which accurate communication can enable clients to cope with change and crisis. Embedded within the theoretical framework based on the work of Bowlby (1973) and Rutter (1981), both of whom focus upon the developmental needs for close fostering relationships, we suggest that health care workers have a role to play in helping clients to re-establish an equilibrium using skilled communication. This can range from practical advice to providing emotional support through the skill of active listening and the Rogerian core conditions of genuineness, acceptance, and empathy.

Chapter 4 deals with issues surrounding the education of health care workers as adult learners. Aspects of learning effective communication skills and identifying methods that are likely to enhance this learning process are addressed. Starting with an acknowledgement that health care workers, as adult learners, require a different educational approach to that of children (Knowles, 1984), we explore the assumption that adults have a desire to be involved in their learning, and also how educators and trainers can encourage this involvement and utilize it in helping people to acquire the knowledge and skills of communication. We emphasize the value of experiential teaching methods over more traditional didactic methods because the high 'action' component of communication skills is complemented by the 'action' learning of experiential approaches. This chapter, therefore, examines the main teaching methods used by the authors, highlighting their advantages and disadvantages. We do not pretend that this list is exhaustive or that the methods used will always be successful. Indeed, our main message to educators and trainers is accurately to identify the needs of the group and match the teaching techniques to those needs, balancing the risks of the method against the benefits of the outcomes.

Part II: The Communication Skills Workshops

Part II of this book provides a series of interconnected workshops intended to guide the user through the skills of effective communication. Each workshop contains a number of exercises relating to specific areas of communication and a specific set of skills. Succeeding workshops offer greater depth and complexity, the emphasis being on the synthesis of the components of communication skills, to enable participants to begin to see communication as a holistic and integrated activity.

Although it is intended that the workshops should be offered sequentially, each is a complete teaching package and can be used as a single session to meet the specific need of a group or when there are constraints on time. However, we do not recommend omitting any of the discussion and reflection times. We also believe that learning is enhanced when it occurs in a group setting, benefiting from divergent views that can challenge personal prejudice and enrich a discussion of the effectiveness or otherwise of interventions. These advantages outweigh the possible pitfalls of group pressures influencing individuals to conform to less effective ways of using communication skills. We suggest that the sequences of exercises and discussions in this part of the book are followed as closely as possible because they are presented in such a way to make a complete and balanced learning experience.

Chapter 5 contains an introductory workshop, which sets the scene for all of the subsequent workshops. It provides an overview of the elements of verbal, nonverbal and active listening skills and offers a series of exercises to give participants an opportunity to sample the skills and feelings associated with these three elements

The next three chapters explore each of these elements in more depth. In Chapter 6, the nonverbal component of communication is examined, with an exploration of the use of nonverbal signals by using role play. This session also initiates participants in the use of video recording as a learning tool. The second part of this workshop focuses on the nonverbal messages used to convey emotions, offering an opportunity for participants to identify cultural and developmental differences in their interpretation via the nonverbal messages being expressed. Chapter 7 presents the workshop examining verbal communication through using role play situations constructed by participants. This is followed by an opportunity to consider the difficulties of using verbal communication techniques accurately to convey information in the absence of a nonverbal component. Chapter 8 offers a workshop on the effective use of active listening, examining this concept from one theoretical perspective that of Watts (1986), and identifying the skills involved. A distinction is made between active and attentive listening by exploring the feelings and thoughts associated with both types of listening as well as the feelings experienced when attention is diverted from the client's concerns.

The next three chapters begin to consolidate and integrate the elements of communication, placing them within the context of a relationship with clients. We have separated the skills of opening interactions, sustaining and controlling interactions, and closing interactions. Chapter 9 focuses on opening interactions, using exercises to explore the ease/difficulty relating to introductions. Following this, role play gives an opportunity to examine openings in more depth. Chapter 10 presents a workshop containing exercises that highlight specific types of intervention that help to sustain an interaction and the affective components of words and behaviours. Also within this workshop are exercises aimed at experiencing the skills and feelings associated with those rare occasions when it is necessary to control an interaction to maintain its therapeutic quality. The specific technique of 'talk-over' is included here. Chapter 11 fittingly ends the series of workshops by examining ending interactions, closing therapeutic relationships, and the consequences for the client of not ending therapeutically.

Setting up Communication Skills Workshops

All the workshops tend to follow the same format. We believe that providing this consistency of approach allays the anxiety of participants and provides a template that facilitators can use to design their own workshops. Below we set out the pattern for workshops.

Introducing a Workshop

The facilitators need to state:

- *Learning outcomes for the workshop*
- *Methods used* Identify the teaching methods to be used, suggesting that full participation will greatly enhance the learning outcomes. Give an outline of what will be required from the participants. Also be explicit about the use of role play and video recording, as these can be difficult for some individuals. Encourage participants to use them but offer those who do not want to take

part the opportunity to participate in other ways (perhaps as observers).

- *Safety* Prepare participants for particular exercises by warning them beforehand to dress appropriately. Soft-soled footwear or socks are preferable for some activities and, for women, trousers may be more comfortable than skirts. Also obtain agreement from participants that personal material divulged during the workshop will not be disclosed outside the group.

- *Time considerations* Let participants know how long the workshop will last and give an indication of the length of particular sections within it. Also make explicit time for breaks to allow participants to reflect on their work and to recuperate from it.

- *Housekeeping issues* Discuss room arrangement, meal venues, and the locations of toilets and telephones. Also make clear where messages can be left.

Conducting a Workshop

When conducting a workshop, it is helpful to follow a consistent format. The workshops in Part II of this book offer a standard structure to enable facilitators to prepare for the exercises and to conduct them consistently. Structuring the workshops at the planning stage allows the facilitators to be more flexible in their implementation. This structure is as follows:

Exercise: Name of Exercise/Warm-up/Game

- *Outcomes*
  Make explicit to participants what are the expected outcomes of the exercise and, if necessary, enable them to make the links with previous exercises and workshops.

- *Configuration*
  Discuss how the group will need to divide to complete the exercise. Ask the members of the group to form themselves into the necessary configuration (pairs, triads, small group or the whole group). Pay attention to those declining to complete the exercise. Also note odd numbers of participants; facilitators should be prepared to participate themselves to make up numbers.

- *Time*
  If necessary, give a rough indication of how long the exercise will take but do not get too concerned about meeting self-imposed deadlines, especially if there is important material being discussed.

- *Materials*
  Indicate what materials the participants will need and tell them what you will provide and what they will need to bring themselves.
- *Process*
  State as clearly as possible what the participants actually have to do. Also identify the facilitator's role. Allow time for clarification but do not be afraid to encourage the participants just to plunge in; experiential work is about experiencing uncertainty and being creative.

De-roling

After any role play exercise, especially one having a high emotional content, it is important that participants should disengage from the role they played and 'ground' themselves back into the reality of the workshop. This helps to reduce the risk of the emotional experiences of the role being displaced and is done by de-roling. A number of exercises are available, but we have found the most effective one is simply to bring all the participants together and invite each person to say who they were in the role play, who they really are now and something that is true about themselves in the here and now (for example, 'I am wearing a blue shirt', or 'It is nearly lunchtime and I am hungry'). While de-roling does not have to be elaborate, it is an important element in providing a safe learning environment.

Evaluating the Workshop

All workshops should be evaluated; this enables both the participants and the facilitators to recognize the positive and negative aspects. Evaluation can take the form of written questionnaires or (of particular value in experiential workshops) immediate verbal feedback. This latter allows both facilitators and participants to examine their own performances and to make available to others the fruits of their reflection. It can also provide facilitators with feedback about their own work and the workshop as a whole. Evaluation can take any form; we provide a standard format below, although we would encourage readers to adapt this to meet their own needs:

- *Outcomes*
  Make explicit that this final part of the workshop is expected to meet the following outcomes:
    Help participants to identify what they liked most and least about the workshop as a whole;

Enable facilitators to identify parts of the workshop that might
need alteration in the future;
Allow time for reflection upon practice and skills acquisition.

- *Configuration*
The whole group seated in a circle.

- *Time*
Fifteen minutes (approximately).

- *Process*
Each member of the group (including the facilitator) in turn
states one thing they liked least about any aspect of the workshop.
This can include facilitation, the material, the exercises, or their
own performance during the day.
Members may 'pass' at their turn but must not justify or respond
to requests for justification of any statement they make.
After each has responded or 'passed', each member in turn states
one thing they liked most about the workshop.

Summary

This chapter has mapped the book's contents, giving an overview
of the links between the theoretical aspects in Part I and the practical
aspects of the workshops in Part II. It has offered a possible
structure for readers to devise their own workshops in relation to
communications or any other skill-related topic. In presenting a
complete skills-based communications curriculum, we do not want
to imply that this is in any way definitive. We would encourage
anyone contemplating devising a teaching session or series of workshops to be creative and free to adapt these workshops and exercises
in whatever way is necessary to help to maximize the learning
experience.

We hope that participating in communication skills training,
either as a facilitator or as a learner, will be stimulating, creative
and enjoyable and, above all, will result in more effective communication with clients.

Chapter 2
Communication in Health Care

Communication is an essential and inevitable feature of human existence. It is not surprising, therefore, that communication takes place in a variety of ways. It can be direct or indirect, conscious or unconscious, overt or covert. We use verbal and nonverbal signals to indicate emotional states, such as grief or happiness, and similarly to give an indication of physical state, such as pain or tiredness. However, they might be used in an attempt to conceal physical or emotional discomfort, although, in most cases, this is difficult (Hargie, 1986). Communication is, of course, also used for specific purposes, such as the conscious transmission of information, as in education, or satisfactorily to achieve a particular outcome, such as when selling something. It is instrumental in developing and forming relationships, which might be beneficial to the individuals involved, although, when used perversely, it could lead to the deliberate and malicious harm of another individual (Heron, 1989). In any event, it would seem that communication is a feature of all living cells (Patton and Griffin, 1974). However, expressions such as: 'He doesn't know how to communicate,' or 'She failed to communicate,' conflict with the view that communication is an inevitable part of life; we must assume that these comments are used figuratively and relate to a frustration of the outcome of communication rather than any inability of the individual. In settings such as health care, where communication is vital and workers can influence the well-being of vulnerable individuals, an opportunity for practitioners to explore and practise these skills is likely to increase the achievement of effective outcomes. Undertaking this exploration involves scrutinizing the components of communication, the context in which they work best, and what elements are most effective.

Channels of Communication

A common way to conceptualize human communication is when two or more people are in contact. This contact consists of a message, an encoding or encryption of the message, a path to transmit, and a means of decoding. The message can be transmitted and received using any of the senses at the disposal of the individuals. It may be reciprocal or unilateral, although even 'one-way' communication channels are still open for an exchange to take place. For example, in face to face contact, nonverbal signals will still be transmitted by the recipient and affect the sender's subsequent message, even though the communication is supposed to be in one direction. This model can be described as an information processing model of communication (Barber, 1988); however, it implies that the procedure is mechanical and is not influenced by other factors that need to be taken into account when examining what may influence its transmission and/or reception.

All individuals' communication with each other will have internal factors, which will influence how a message is sent or received. These include such things as beliefs, intended goals, physical and emotional states, and the perception of others' influence, role, status or personality, as well as assumptions about a number of factors within the communication, such as their perceptions of the friendliness of the other parties. External factors that may affect communication include environmental, social, biological, psychological and economic influences.

However, the division between the internal and external factors that influence communication is an artificial one, as each influences the other. For example, the internal factor of child rearing beliefs in parents will have an effect upon the parents' behaviour towards the child and subsequently the child's behaviour in the outside world (Mussen et al. 1990). By the same token, external factors of an individual's life can influence their internal world. A classic example of this is in a study by Brown and Harris (1978), in which they identified four social factors that have the ability to precipitate depression in some women. Therefore, when using communication therapeutically, it is prudent that health care workers should recognize this mix of internal and external influences. Figure 2.1 offers a method of conceptualizing message transmission and reception, which takes account of the influence of internal and external factors. For a more comprehensive description of these processes, it is suggested that the reader should look at any of the following: Beck et al. (1988); Bradley and Edinberg (1990); Ellis and Beattie (1986); Hargie (1986); Porritt (1990); Sundeen et al. (1989).

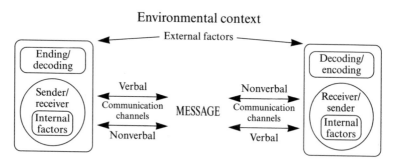

Figure 2.1 Message transmission and reception

Components of Communication

While internal and external factors are important influences upon the process, the components of communication have attracted much attention and analysis. There have been various descriptions of the components, including: a psycholinguistic structure (Chomsky, 1965; Garnham, 1985; Green, 1987; Slobin, 1979); an interpersonal/interactional function (Argyle, 1983; Egan, 1990a; Hargie, 1986; Heron, 1989; Nelson-Jones, 1982; Sundeen *et al.* 1989; Trower *et al.* 1978); and a developmental/acquisitional role (Cromer, 1991; Mussen *et al.* 1990; Sutherland, 1992; Vygotsky, 1962). However, it can also be beneficial to examine communication via the systems used and their interrelatedness as demonstrated by Ellis and Beattie (1986) (Figure 2.2).

In describing the constituents of these systems, Ellis and Beattie (1986) have suggested that one of the communication systems is verbal and the other nonverbal. Verbal communication contains words, phrases and sentences. This would include the techniques of paraphrasing, reflecting feelings, immediacy, open questions, probing questions and clarifying questions, and also enabling the exchange of information, the clarification of issues, the demonstration of understanding, and the offering of support and direction. Nonverbal communication consists of four elements. First, there is a prosodic system, which helps to give meaning to the words used by identifying the intonation and rhythm of a verbal utterance, as well as placing pauses in positions that give the utterance its most effective emphasis. Secondly, there is a paralinguistic system, which consists of vocal but nonverbal expressions (such as 'mmm' and 'uh huh'). Thirdly, there is a kinesic system, which consists of what is usually considered 'body

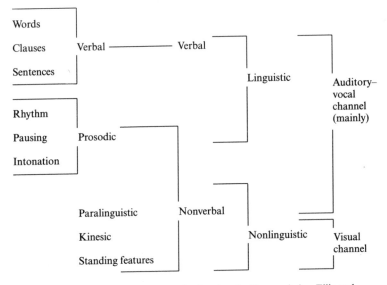

Figure 2.2 Systems of human communication (used with permission Ellis and Beattie, 1986)

language' (gestures, facial expressions, etc.), which is so important in expressing emotion, communicating interpersonal attitudes, and accompanying and supporting speech, self-presentation and rituals (Argyle, 1988). Finally, Ellis and Beattie (1986) suggest standing features as a component of nonverbal communication. These include elements such as the communicator's appearance (i.e. clothes, adornments, scent, etc.). They also identify proxemics, which include interpersonal and personal space, and touch as other important aspects of communication.

Within health care settings, we suggest that listening is an important component in the development and maintenance of a therapeutic relationship (Egan, 1990a; Nelson-Jones, 1982). However, listening is not simply the passive reception of the client's communication but is a skill arising from the active combination of verbal and nonverbal communication systems. Active listening, therefore, can be understood as the bridge between verbal and nonverbal communication because it uses both of these, enabling the health care worker to listen to the manifest and latent content of what is being said (Watts, 1986), and respond appropriately to the client's message. Figure 2.3 shows a representation of active

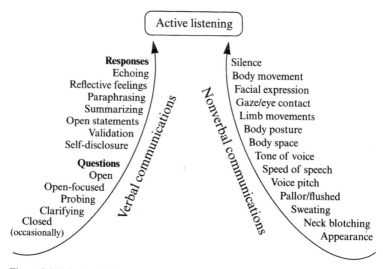

Figure 2.3 Relationship between active listening and verbal/nonverbal communications

listening through the relationship between verbal and nonverbal communication.

Effective Communication in Health Care

It is our contention that health care is underpinned by effective communication. However, this begs the question of how effective communication can be identified, and who decides whether or not it has been effective. In answering this question it is necessary to distinguish between process and outcome. It is an underlying theme of this book that the client should take part in the definition of the effectiveness of the outcome of communication. It must be recognized that under specific, and limited, circumstances, such as when a person is in danger of self-harm, either deliberately or inadvertently, the health care worker may have to be prescriptive. However, generally effective communication will be promoted when there is a mutual assessment regarding its effectiveness between the health care worker and the client.

A classic study within the nursing profession that demonstrates the efficacy of communication and co-operation in patient care is that of Hayward (1975). He found that patients offered specific information about the level of discomfort and what procedures they might expect prior to undergoing operations, resulted in the patients experiencing much less postoperative pain and a faster recovery than patients not given such information. Similarly, in a study of patients undergoing surgery for gynaecological cancer, Corney *et al.* (1992) found that clients actively sought postoperative information from nursing staff concerning a variety of issues, from practical to sexual relationships. These studies demonstrate how active collaboration with and involvement of clients in elements of their care tends to be well received by clients and can markedly contribute to an improvement in their health.

The effectiveness of communication should also be judged in terms of the process. We have suggested earlier that listening skills are a central feature of communication and that it is an active process combining verbal and nonverbal communication systems. In two studies by Honeycutt and Worobey (1987) concerning the impressions of communication effectiveness, the use of listening skills by nurses was found to be an important factor in effective communication with patients, irrespective of the stage of the nurse–patient relationship. They also found that attentiveness was an important factor in patients' perceptions, of effective communication. In order for someone to be identified as being attentive, it is necessary for them to use appropriate nonverbal skills including body posture, facial expression and eye contact (Argyle, 1983). Egan (1990a) described a series of nonverbal behaviours that tended to signal attentiveness. These can be remembered by the acronym SOLER, which stands for Sitting squarely, Open posture with the client, Leaning forward slightly, Eye contact, and maintaining a Relaxed position. Health care workers who use these behaviours are more likely to be perceived as attentive and sympathetic by their clients, although Hermansson *et al.* (1988) noted that timing was important in using these skills and, for example, leaning forward at an inappropriate time could reduce intensity and respect in the interaction. Therefore, health care workers need to respond appropriately to the subtle cues they receive from their clients and be prepared to match their own behaviour to that of the client in order to maintain an equilibrium and a level of mutuality in the interaction taking place. Some cues that may be observed by the health care worker in the course of an interaction will include the level of skin pallor, which could be indicative of client distress, or excess limb movement, which might indicate anxiety. Changes in the muscles around the eyes can also be detected and may signify levels of fear or anger (Matsumoto, 1989). Indications of distress, insecurity and conflict may also be detected in the client's rhythm, pausing or intonation (Smith and Clark, 1993). The health care worker might need explicitly to investigate the meaning of such signals with the client.

Clients are more likely to view the health care worker as an effective communicator when the language used in the interaction is familiar and jargon free. While technical terms might need to be used for the sake of accuracy in explaining a situation or procedure to a client, it is the responsibility of the health care worker to explain these terms in a clear, familiar and nonpatronizing way. To do this might involve the health care worker in learning new language skills, such as when working with ethnic minorities or people with hearing impairments. For example, Haley and Dowd (1988) found that deaf adolescents who were adept at sign language rated counsellors (whether hearing impaired or not) as being more influential, effective and empathic if they used sign language rather than written messages or an interpreter. It thus seems that, in order for effective communication to take place, health care workers need to attend to the client's, as well as to their own, verbal and nonverbal messages. They also need to acknowledge the context within which the interaction is taking place and how that might affect either their own or the client's internal environment.

Summary

As stated earlier, communication is an inevitable part of existence; it is not unique to humans. It can be conceptualized as a series of components that require a message, a transmitter, a receiver and a channel for transmission. The elements can be broadly categorized into verbal and nonverbal components; both of these combine in the skill of active listening, which is a cornerstone of effective communication in health care settings. Effective communication needs to be judged in terms of both the outcome of the communication (whether the interaction achieved what was intended) and the process (whether the communication was accurate, empathic and fostered a helping, therapeutic relationship between the client and the health care worker). We suggest that the effectiveness of communication, whether viewed in terms of process or outcome, is something that must be judged by both health care worker and client.

For a client to be able to collaborate in the relationship and to be able to state his or her own health care needs requires the development of a safe environment in which a client can disclose and discuss anxiety-provoking issues (Minardi and Riley, 1988). The provision of a psychologically safe environment where clients can discuss intimate material and develop a sense of trust in the health care worker is the subject of the next chapter.

Chapter 3

Psychological Safety Using Skilled Communication

The experience of illness or disability is disturbing for any individual, not merely because of pain or loss of function, but also because it challenges the concept of the self as a fully functioning and whole person. Similarly, the process of learning new skills as a health care worker, such as those involving communication, may require giving up cherished preconceptions of already being a proficient, skilful carer and communicator. These challenges to the person's unique view of self often generate anxiety. Coping with this might result in developing avoidance strategies, which, while reducing anxiety, can prevent change, development and the growth of the individual.

In this situation, both the health care worker and the client have something in common: the need to feel safe as they face the anxiety brought about by change and ultimately having to accept a new view of themselves that incorporates the process and outcome of change. Emphasizing the affinity between carer and client is a significant step towards enhancing the understanding and empathy that must be present in any successful caring relationship. Therefore, when facilitating communication skill development in psychologically safe conditions, not only will health care workers assimilate the knowledge, skills and attitudes necessary to become competent but they will also begin to provide the elements of psychological and physical safety for their clients.

There are a number of ways in which a person's perception of safety, both physical and psychological, can be enhanced; this chapter will explore some of these. This will include an examination of commonly used coping mechanisms, and how health care workers can provide the environmental and emotional conditions to promote effective coping in their clients.

Table 3.1 Constituents of psychological safety (after Rutter, 1981)

- The opportunity to develop enduring bonds within stable and stimulating relationships
- Nourishment
- Care and protection
- Role models
- Play and conversation
- Boundaries within which these can be provided

Psychological Safety

To understand the concept of psychological safety in relationships between adults we must turn to the theories of development of the personality in childhood. The development of the unique 'self' is a continuing process involving the evolution of intellectual and emotional attributes, the processing of external information via the senses, and the presence of social influences, all of which enable growth and development of the person. This last element is particularly important given that the failure to develop warm and continuing attachments in childhood tends to decrease the possibility of developing healthy relationships when older (Bowlby, 1973). Although there is much debate about the constituents of significant attachments, the developing child generally needs love and the opportunity to build enduring bonds within stable and stimulating relationships (Rutter, 1981). Additionally, the growing child needs nourishment, care and protection, role models, play and conversation, and, above all, boundaries within which these can be provided (Table 3.1). In other words, the developing person needs conditions conducive to feeling safe and secure on the journey from childhood to adulthood.

Adults are no different to developing children in needing to feel safe and protected. An absence of the above elements can make the world a dangerous and unsafe place for a person, and, although this perception of risk does not necessarily mean that there will be irreparable damage, it inevitably brings distress, some of which may persist over long periods. This distress can take the form of anger and resentment, or hopelessness, despair and depression, and, finally, disengagement, indifference and detachment. For some people this despair may become an enduring element of his or her personality, not necessarily disrupting the individual's life totally but colouring and influencing the person's experiences and making the subjective view of themselves and those around them less secure. Conversely,

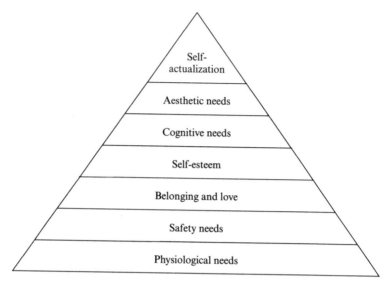

Figure 3.1 Maslow's hierarchy of needs (after Maslow, 1970)

an individual (be they adult or child) will tend to grow as an assured, confident, self-possessed and secure person when provided with enough of those elements that enhance psychological safety.

The Concept of the Self and Change

To be human is to experience change. All of life involves confronting change as part of a natural cycle in which birth, childhood, adolescence, adulthood, parenthood, middle age, old age and, ultimately, death, bring their own challenges that people may respond to and use for developing and growing in ways that help to affirm themselves as unique individuals. These critical periods of change are not simply biological but also involve the individual interacting with others and completing certain tasks as he or she develops (Erikson, 1969). Coping with change requires certain conditions to be met. Maslow suggests that all humans have a 'hierarchy of needs' (Figure 3.1). This includes basic needs for sustenance, safety and love and belonging, which must be met before individuals can value themselves and begin to 'self-actualize' (i.e. find self-fulfilment and realize their true potential) (Maslow, 1970). Thus, if it is assumed that change is a feature of all our lives, then our experiences of being loved and cared for – or the absence of these conditions – will significantly affect the way we view ourselves as individuals and motivate ourselves to fulfil our unique potential.

Crisis and Coping

Among the changes some people face is the experience of ill health. This is critical because it brings not only the possibility of pain and loss of function but also changes in the concept of the self as a whole person. This loss of a sense of wholeness and health is often a significant moment of risk and crisis to an individual, which can either stimulate personal inner strengths and resources to resolve or accommodate the change, or can provoke anxiety, upset and crisis. If perceived as a crisis, it may be understood as an experience of loss or a challenge that outstrips an individual's ability to cope, implying an essentially subjective experience.

Physiologically, humans react to crisis by releasing adrenaline and preparing to fight or flee. However, this reaction can only be sustained for a few minutes and, consequently, if the experience continues, further coping mechanisms are invoked to survive the stress. These may directly focus on the causes of the crisis and attempt to reduce the threat, for example by stopping smoking and taking more exercise to reduce the risk of high blood pressure. Conversely, persons may use indirect mechanisms to reduce their anxiety or to change their perception of the problem. This may include adaptive strategies like learning to relax or talking over fears and worries with someone. On the other hand, people sometimes use maladaptive strategies to cope with a crisis, emphasizing specific defence mechanisms such as denial ('I'll never have a heart attack') or rationalization ('I don't need to give up smoking; my father smoked 20 a day for 40 years'). Brown and Pedder (1991) describe a number of defence mechanisms, which they suggest are commonly used to protect against anxiety and what they term 'psychic pain'. These include:

- *Repression* The ignoring (suppression) of inconvenient or unacceptable thoughts or the consigning (repression) of disagreeable feelings into the unconscious;
- *Denial* The forgetting or rejection of an unpleasant external event (e.g. denying the death of a loved one);
- *Projection* Attributing to or behaving as though other people contain feelings or attributes that in fact belong to us;

- *Reaction formation* Obscuring unacceptable traits in ourselves by adopting an opposite extreme of behaviour;
- *Rationalization* Consciously justifying an unconscious desire or impulse;
- *Conversion* The transformation of unacceptable feelings into physical symptoms;
- *Displacement* Deflecting strong feelings from the true source to someone or somewhere less threatening;
- *Regression* Coping with misfortune by reverting to more childlike or dependent ways of coping;
- *Sublimation* The expression of unconscious desires or motives in modified, socially acceptable ways.

Coping mechanisms such as these may be continued over a long period and essentially help a person to deal with anxiety, although they may not be useful or effective for the longer term survival of the person (i.e. some coping mechanisms can be damaging).

Coping with Ill Health

Ill health challenges everyone's ability to cope. In the course of their professional lives, health care workers will encounter people who are attempting to cope with illness by employing a variety of strategies or coping mechanisms, some of which will be more successful than others. There is a great deal of evidence to suggest that the more easily clients cope with stress, the less likely they are to become ill and, if they do, the more likely they are to recover (Bond, 1971; Rachman and Philips, 1975; Sternbach, 1968). As we discussed earlier, how people deal with stress, including ill health, will be shaped by childhood influences. Added to this is the importance of how much control they feel they have over their circumstances and the extent to which they perceive they have support. Successful coping with ill health demands that people should either overcome illnesses or adapt to the changes they may bring.

Achieving this requires clients to feel that they have some control over the situation and to sense that they are supported as they come to terms with the changes brought about by the loss of health and the attempt to regain it. Wills and Langner (1980) suggest that there are a number of elements that might enable people to perceive themselves as being supported and thus be able to cope with ill health. These include coping modelled by family and friends, assistance in solving problems, guidance, perceived control over circumstances,

Table 3.2 A model for providing safety and support through skilled communication

---

Enabling family and friends to model successful coping strategies
Offering direct assistance in solving problems
Giving appropriate guidance
Encouraging perceptions of control over circumstances
Making sure appropriate information is available
Fostering security and enhanced self-esteem

---

the availability of information and security, and enhanced self-esteem (Table 3.2).

The health care worker who can provide these elements will be enabling clients to take some control and thereby go some way towards effectively meeting the challenge of ill health.

Communicating Emotional Support

Communicating support and developing a safe and sensitive relationship requires a degree of skilful communication. The health care worker occupies a special position in relation to his or her client, being neither relative nor friend, and yet needing to avoid supplanting the warmth, closeness and friendship offered by family and friends. To do this successfully demands the skill to develop close and confiding relationships that do not overpower the client's capacity to cope.

Carl Rogers (1961) recognized the importance of developing relationships as a means of change, and summarized this in the now famous phrase: 'If I can provide a certain type of relationship, the other person will discover within himself the capacity to use that relationship for growth, and change and personality development will occur' (p. 33).

Rogers went on to propose a number of requirements or conditions that are at the heart of a helping relationship. He suggested that there are three fundamental characteristics that a helper needs to demonstrate within a relationship and that are necessary to enable the person being helped to change and develop: genuineness, empathy and acceptance.

Genuineness

Genuineness is the condition in which a helper in the relationship is behaving (and is perceived as behaving) in a way that reflects and constantly matches the inner feelings that that person has about the individual with whom he or she is working. This congruence between inner and outer selves enables health care workers to be honest and spontaneous with their clients, accepting and expressing both positive and negative feelings. This will facilitate frank and sincere communication between helpers and clients.

Genuineness, sometimes called realness or authenticity, enables the client to see that the person helping them is a real and authentic person rather than simply a professional therapist offering an impersonal service. It involves the helper in being willing to disclose his or her thoughts and feelings in a forthright yet caring manner in order to enable the client to feel safe enough to talk equally candidly about personal problems and difficulties. The helper, expressing a willingness to be known not just as a helper but as a real and genuine person, will find that the client will be encouraged to respond similarly. In other words, disclosure begets disclosure.

Being genuine and congruent does not mean that the helper can have licence to say whatever is on his or her mind. For example, to indicate to the client that he or she is annoying or unhelpful could be insulting and counter-productive. Similarly, genuineness is not about the helper having an arena in which to talk about him- or herself. To do so would risk focusing more upon the helper's feelings than upon the client's. As the main intention of communication is to enable clients to convey their own thoughts and feelings, the helper must select from the inevitable variety of authentic feelings and thoughts that he or she will have about the clients, and use those that are most relevant, persistent and striking with regard to the client situation (Mearns and Thorne, 1988).

An example of genuineness being used to strengthen and deepen a helping relationship might be when a health care worker becomes aware of an inner sense of frustration with a client who incessantly seeks reassurance that he or she is making progress or getting better. The health care worker might address this feeling in the course of a conversation in the following way.

> *Worker* Every time we meet you ask me if you are going to get better, and it's really hard for me to know how to reply to you in a way that is helpful.
>
> *Client* I'm sorry. It's just that I really don't think I'm getting any better.
>
> *Worker* I think you're sounding really sorry for yourself now. . . .
> That wasn't a very nice thing for me to say. I guess that part of me wants to help you but it feels as though I'm being blocked and that's really frustrating.

Client That's all right. I know you are doing your best and you want to help. It's just that I get really frightened that there won't be anyone like you there when I go home.

Worker It sounds almost as though you don't want to go home. . . .

In this example, the health care worker has addressed a persistent problem in the helping relationship and in the course of this reacts to the client, but then follows this up by reflecting openly upon the remark and then going on to make plain his or her underlying thoughts and feelings brought about by the client's behaviour. This enables the client to access the feeling of anxiety about isolation and vulnerability, which the health care worker can then follow.

Empathy

The core condition of empathy refers to the ability to sense how a person is feeling and reacting, and to communicate that to the person. Being empathic also involves possessing personal attributes of sensibility and sensitivity to others and an ability to convey this to them. Therefore it is both a personal attribute and a skill.

Empathy as a personal attribute of the health care worker involves 'being with' the other person in a relationship, acknowledging and prizing the existence of the other. It is a mode of human contact in which the health care worker can respond to clients 'as if' he or she were that other person but without losing the sense of his or her own self. Empathy occurs when one person acknowledges another's internal frame of reference, and, paradoxically, thereby recognizes the separateness and uniqueness of that other person. Rogers (1980) describes this 'being with' as entering the private world of the client and being responsive to changing meanings within the client and to the emotions that he or she is experiencing, without making judgements.

Empathy also requires a communication process that involves a series of skills enabling the client's perceptual world, having been grasped, to be reflected back to the client, thereby signalling a comprehension and sharing of this inner world. These skills include a variety of verbal and nonverbal interventions, which will be focused upon in the second part of this book.

Empathy needs to be clearly distinguished from sympathy. The former arises from a sensitivity to another person's perceptions, understanding and feelings, leading to a willingness to bear witness to that person's distress and to encourage and validate his or her attempts to manage it. Sympathy, on the other hand, often originates from within the perceiver as a desire only to perceive someone else's suffering from the perceiver's perspective, rather than that of the person in distress. While this is not necessarily a negative sentiment, it is more likely to lead towards finding solutions for the client that are based upon the health care worker's own needs rather than those of the client. This 'doing unto' rather than 'doing with' clients can discline them from finding their own ways of coping.

An example of an empathetic approach is given in the following example, in which a health care worker encounters a client sitting in front of an uneaten meal:

Worker You don't seem to have eaten anything.

Client I'm not hungry.

Worker Not hungry at all? Or just not wanting to eat what's here?

Client I'm not sure what you mean. . . .

Worker I wonder if you are telling me that you don't like being in a position where other people are bringing you food.

Client I suppose I've been used to looking after myself for a long time.

In this example, the health care worker tried to put him- or herself in the shoes of the client by focusing not simply upon the physiological need for nourishment but on the client's need for self-esteem, which may be being damaged by an enforced dependency. This level of sensing often happens intuitively and requires a deep understanding of the client and a willingness to take a risk in moving from the more concrete world of providing for bodily needs into the abstract world of the emotions.

Unconditional Positive Regard

Sometimes referred to as the quality of acceptance or nonpossessive warmth, unconditional positive regard is the third of Rogers' core conditions, which, when communicated to a client, will help to sustain a warm and supportive relationship. Rogers himself described this attribute as the 'prizing' of the person to convey the sense of warmth and respect that is required. The client will bring to a helping relationship a variety of thoughts, feelings, behaviours and attitudes, some of which may be a central and defining part of the person, and others that may be a reaction to the health problems they are enduring. The health care worker wanting to overcome barriers to developing a relationship will need to be tolerant, respectful and accepting of the person as he or she is. The underlying aim is to affirm the worth of the individual and what that person brings to the relationship or the situation.

For health care workers, the most difficult aspect of this condition will be the need for unconditionality. Many relationships in everyday life are conditional, with respect and acceptance coming only when we meet certain conditions, like being pleasant or helpful. It may not be particularly easy for health care workers to make the transition into a health care setting where they will inevitably meet situations that challenge the ability to provide an unqualified acceptance of an individual. This may be because the thoughts, feelings, behaviours and attitudes of the client get in the way of acceptance. For example, it can be very hard to respect a client who is abusive or violent. In this case, unconditional regard does not mean that behaviour that is harmful or injurious to others (or to the client's own person) should be accepted, and firm limits regarding the consequences of a particular behaviour may need to be made explicit. However, in doing so, health care workers need to attempt to reject the behaviour of an individual without rejecting the person. The following example may help to illuminate this difficult concept.

> *Client* Look, I've been waiting 40 minutes and I still haven't seen the doctor. If you don't go and find him right now, I'll bust the place up.
>
> *Worker* I can see you are very angry, and I want you to get seen as soon as possible. I know that...
>
> *Client* Don't tell me what you know, just get the doctor before I smash the place up.
>
> *Worker* I'm willing to go and see what the delay is all about but if you smash the place up I'm worried that you may not get seen at all. If you tell me where you are sitting, I'll go right now and find out what is happening and come straight back to you. Would that help?

In that very difficult situation the health care worker avoided retaliating with anger and stayed focused upon the client and his (or her) needs, offering to help the client and indirectly suggesting that the client should return to the waiting area. The final checking out with the client implies that the angry feelings have not precluded the client from being consulted.

Summary

Ill health may cause individuals to reappraise their view of themselves and perhaps to cease to view themselves as whole and functioning people. This change in view tends to be anxiety provoking, and coping with this 'new identity', be it temporary or permanent, requires the security of a safe and nurturing relationship.

This need stems from childhood in which, to develop as functioning and coping human beings we require the opportunity to build stable and stimulating relationships that can be used as a platform for growth and change. Alongside this we have other requirements, which form a hierarchy of needs and include physiological and safety needs together with a sense of belonging and love. When these are met, then an individual can develop self-esteem, which leads to the ability to seek those things that meet the person's cognitive and aesthetic needs. The presence of these are vital to our development as fully functioning humans.

In times of crisis, individuals may adopt a number of psychological strategies or defence mechanisms to cope with anxiety. These include such things as repression, denial, projection, conversion and regression. Recognizing these is a vital task for health care workers. In addition, psychological safety will be enhanced when a number of other client conditions are met, including: enabling family and friends to help; offering direct assistance, information and appropriate guidance; encouraging positive perceptions of control over circumstances; and fostering security and enhanced self-esteem. This last condition can be met by health care workers if they are able to use communication skills effectively to convey genuine, empathic and unconditional acceptance in their relationships with clients.

Thus, as suggested earlier in this chapter, a process of learning can be of benefit to health care workers in helping them to strengthen their communication skills and provide the above conditions to create psychological safety for clients. The next chapter examines ways in which this process may be addressed.

Chapter 4

Facilitating the Acquisition of Skilled Communications

We have suggested that competent communication is an essential aspect of health care, enabling information to be given and received, helping the client to feel safe enough within a client–care giver relationship to explore emotional and psychological elements that may affect health. This raises the question of how health care workers might acquire the skills of communication. One traditional response within health care settings is that there is no need to 'acquire' them, as they are a natural part of being human and are developed from childhood. This view has support from theorists such as the psycholinguist Naom Chomsky (1965), who suggests language learning and speech acquisition are innate and that the process begins within the first months of life (Mussen *et al.* 1990; Sutherland, 1992). Conversely, recent research suggests that education does have an effect on the ability of psychiatric nurses to identify emotions from the nonverbal communication of facial expression (Minardi, 1995), which implies that training can enhance the ability of health care workers to interact more effectively with clients. It should be recognized that communication may not be effective in a health care setting because individuals or organizations are unsure about whether communication skills are needed; there is little clarity about what makes communication effective, and the manner in which communication skills training is presented does not meet the needs of individuals who *do* recognize that they would benefit from training (Fielding and Llewelyn, 1987). However, we suggest that to enhance our innate ability to communicate and use that communication skilfully – in the right form, with the right delivery, at the right time, and with the right people – requires an educational process to facilitate the acquisition of skilled communication rather than a reliance solely upon the natural maturation of innate mechanisms.

This chapter will address the influence we believe learning can have on the development of effective communication skills. It will give a brief description of adult learning and address how skills in communication and its associated concepts might be acquired. Finally, there will be a discussion of the concept of experiential learning and an overview of the main teaching methods that we have employed in the communication skills workshops.

Overview of Adult Learning

Education can be viewed as an activity aimed at increasing an individual's intellectual capacity, character and potential, reasoning, understanding, skill development, morals, and social behaviour (Peters, 1963, 1966). This would include development in the cognitive, perceptual, and psychomotor domains (Pfeiffer, 1985). Therefore, the process of learning will alter an individual's skills, emotions, attitudes, and/or beliefs, as well as knowledge; this alteration may occur consciously or unconsciously. Jarvis (1988), who presumes that learning happens consciously in a planned way suggests that, 'Education may now be defined as any planned series of incidents, having a humanistic basis, directed towards the participants learning and understanding' (p. 26). However, learning may also take place via unplanned experiences and at an unconscious level by, for example, observing and internalizing the behaviour of another person (Bandura, 1977). Such diversity makes education difficult to define (Peters, 1966), but this has not deterred theorists such as Gagne (1985) from proposing that,

> A learning occurrence, then, takes place when the stimulus situation together with the contents of memory affect the student in such a way that his or her performance changes from a time before being in that situation to a time after being in it. The change in performance leads to the conclusion that learning has occurred (p. 4).

It would seem from this that the important factor in education is change and that this process happens with all living organisms (Walker, 1987). Learning through change is consequently a process that, in humans, is unlikely to be limited by age, gender, race or beliefs. Furthermore, learning does not end after a formal, statutory period, and does not take place only in institutions such as universities, but continues, in a variety of forms, throughout life. As Ausubel (1985) puts it, 'education does not end when students leave school' (p. 71). However, he goes on to suggest that individuals need to be taught to learn by themselves, which assumes that learning is a skill and that learning how to learn needs to be 'taught' early to enable it to be continued as adults.

This conflicts with the view that adult learning ('andragogy' is a term coined by Knowles to represent this concept) occurs because adults are self-directed and self-motivated, they have accumulated a considerable reservoir of experience that can assist their learning and become a resource for it. They have a readiness to learn, especially in the problem areas with which they are confronted, and, as a result, they are likely to have an inner desire to learn (Knowles, 1984). Additionally, although adults are likely to want to learn complex skills and gain knowledge for pragmatic reasons, such as solving particular problems with which they are confronted in the working situation, they might also do so for more esoteric reasons, perhaps solely because a subject holds intrinsic interest for them. Whatever the reason, the assumption is that adults will learn when the 'time is right', in subjects in which they are intrinsically or extrinsically motivated, and regardless of whether or how well they have been 'taught' how to learn, although this latter factor would undoubtedly improve the effectiveness of the learning process for individuals.

Knowles' (1984) work acknowledges the influence of the philosopher and educationalist John Dewey (Jarvis, 1988). It recognizes that adult learning benefits from being facilitated rather than didactically presented and will be more likely to happen when the learner's intrinsic motivation is utilized. It also recognizes that education is internally driven, regardless of prior experiences and usually when the individual is ready for learning to occur. It also legitimizes experience in helping adults to learn, which is an important encouraging factor. Thus, strategies that acknowledge the experience and independence of adults, such as contract learning, will reinforce the self-directing role of adults as learners.

Knowles' (1984) concept of andragogy, however, is not without its critics. There is little evidence of the assumption that children and adults learn differently, or whether adults can be assumed to be an homogeneous group and can therefore be placed into a single category for learning purposes. It has been suggested rather frivolously that, since there are some differences between the ways men and women learn, we might therefore 'adopt the term "gynagogy" to describe the education of women' (Darbyshire, 1993: p. 332). However, the important point made by Jarvis (1988) is that, while andragogy is not a theory of adult learning, it has had a strong influence on how adults are taught, especially because of a recognition of the unique qualities of adults as learners, such as their past experiences and overall self-directedness. Therefore, if adults learn in ways that harness their strengths, it is important that facilitators should support and encourage this process while recognizing that there are differences in how and what people learn.

Learning the Skills and Concepts of Communication

As with any other skill, learning to be a good communicator requires an understanding of the different components of communication and the connections between them. This enables the complexities of the skill of communication to be grasped and provides a convenient design for teaching the overall skill. The strategy of limiting learning to each component of the skill in sequence before attempting to perform the whole skill is known as 'serial' learning. It contrasts with the strategy in which the learner attempts the whole skill then works on the parts that require further practice before undertaking the whole skill again (known as 'whole-part-whole' learning). Lovell (1982) has suggested that skills with a high level of organization are best taught using the whole-part-whole method, while skills that are overall of high complexity, with each part not being particularly demanding, are more effectively taught using the serial method. Since communication skills fit both of these criteria, it is more useful that they are taught using a combination of these strategies.

To enable individuals to develop psychomotor, affective, perceptual and cognitive skills requires the provision of a number of elements. These include demonstrations of the skill or its components, the opportunity to practice, and feedback on the results of that practice. Subsequent practice and feedback are needed to increase the learner's competence. Alongside these elements must be the opportunity for the learner to develop a knowledge base relating to the skill. A theoretical input will allow the learner to adapt the skills they have learned when confronted with novel situations. This is of particular importance in health care settings where the complexities of communication are immense and the health care worker must be able to generalize the learning and communicate in response to the needs of the client rather than in a mechanistic manner. Potentially, one of the most constructive ways to accomplish this is by using experiential learning techniques in which the cognitive, behavioural, affective, perceptual and attitudinal components of a subject are explored, cultivated and internalized by the learner.

Experiential Learning and Communication Skills

What does experiential learning involve? The answer to this seemingly simple question has been recounted in a number of sources (see e.g. Burnard, 1989b, 1990; Minton, 1991; Pfeiffer, 1985; Quinn,

1995). The concept also seems straightforward to define, as offered by Pfeiffer (1985): 'Experiential learning occurs when a person engages in some activity, looks back at the activity critically, abstracts some useful insights from the analysis, and puts the result to work' (p. 3). This is a fairly succinct definition and one that does not immediately raise controversy. However, how can one account for the statements by Henry (1989) that, 'Both the experiential theorist and educational practitioner seem to agree on what experiential learning is not,' (p. 27) and, 'There is less agreement on an appropriate positive definition of the term' (p. 28). Consistent with this, in a study involving nurse educationalists, Burnard (1989a) was offered six different ways of defining experiential learning, with four subjects expressing difficulty in proposing any kind of definition.

These difficulties, however, need not impede individuals from recognizing that experiential learning relates, in some way, to their own experience and, as a result of that experience, learning *for that individual* occurs. In order for this learning to occur, it is important that the individual, or group, reflects upon the experience and, if appropriate, alters any subsequent actions. This view is congruous with what Schön (1983) has identified as 'reflection-in-action'. He suggests that practitioners reflect upon their practice while it is occurring and make relevant adjustments as a result. He also points out that the reflection can be *post hoc* (i.e. taking place after the event but still influencing the future actions of the practitioner). These two aspects of reflection are integrated in the forms of experiential learning categorized by Burnard (1990) as learning *through* experience and learning *from* experience. The former he suggests is a result of something being experienced in the present, but the individual (or group) has been primed to 'reflect-in-action' upon the experience as it is occurring, resulting in a learning process. The latter occurs after an experience has taken place and relies solely upon the individual exploring various aspects of the experience, that person's part in it, and how changes can be generated from the result.

From what has been described thus far, rather than offer an all encompassing definition of experiential learning, it seems more appropriate to identify some of its most salient components. First and most important is that experiential learning should contain an experience that embraces knowledge, skills or both, and also contain the standard that is expected to be attained. Secondly, that experience must be retained by being brought into the individual's consciousness, although, it is also possible for vicarious learning to occur at an unconscious level (Bandura, 1977).

The third element of experiential learning is the necessity to reflect upon the experience. This reflection can take many forms, for example, individually or in groups, written or verbally, and using a structured or an unstructured format. Unless this takes place, it is unlikely that learning will occur. Even in vicarious learning, it is extremely likely that at some point the practitioner will reflect upon what he or she is doing, from where that may have derived, and how it has affected that individual's practice. The fourth element is that the learner, in order to benefit from the experience and the reflection, must have an opportunity to practise, test or experiment with the new concepts. In other words, the learner needs to 'have a go' with the new knowledge or skill gained. The final element is revisiting the experience with a different, more acute awareness of the original experience. Thus, the four elements to experiential learning are: the experience, reflections, action and revisiting the experience. These elements have been described in a number of ways (see Burnard, 1990; Henry, 1989; Kolb and Fry, 1975; Pfeiffer, 1985) that highlight a circular and continuously progressive movement in effective learning, which is an important conceptualization in the learning of competent communication skills.

Experiential learning based on action orientated teaching methods and learner participation has the effect of increasing learning that relates to skills and personal development (Pfeiffer, 1985; Townend, 1985). It has been recognized that teaching techniques that encourage activity change maintain learner attention and motivation (Minton, 1991). Therefore, experiential teaching methods, which are based on action and support a regular but flexible change in learning activities, seem to be more effective than passive/didactic methods in helping people to learn effective communication skills.

Many teaching techniques can be described as experiential. Henry (1989) proposes seven categories (personal development, social change, nontraditional learning, prior learning, work experience, learning by doing, and problem-based learning) within the area of experiential learning, under which are approximately 50 specific methods, including activities as diverse as role play and keeping a personal diary. This would afford any facilitator of experiential learning a wide choice of methods limited only by the group's, the teacher's and the organization's expectations, and practicalities such as the number of participants, venue, topic area, resources available, and skills of the facilitator. The next section offers an overview of those teaching techniques employed in the workshops to be found in Part II of this book. For further information, the reader is referred to Burnard (1989b, 1990), Lovell (1982), Minton (1991), Pfeiffer (1985), Priestly *et al.* (1978), Quinn (1995), and Warner Weil and McGill (1989).

Experiential Learning Methods

The techniques used in the workshops set out in Part II of this book can be divided into five categories: group work, individual work, exercises, structured experiences, and role play. These are broad categories and there is inevitably substantial overlap. For example, structured experiences are exercises that often involve group work, but exercises do not have to be structured. The main purpose of this classification is to identify the most salient aspects of each technique to assist participants and facilitators to decide which might be most useful.

Group Work

Jaques (1984) has posited that groups are an important educational medium and serve the function of pooling resources, sharing ideas, and offering mutual support. Group work can take a number of forms within a session, from a whole group discussion to small subgroups of any number. Large groups for discussion after an exercise or role play can enable participants to reflect upon their experience (a vital ingredient to enabling learning from experience). Small groups can be used to focus on a specific task; they can be used as a step to the generation of new ideas, and can be useful at the beginning of experiential learning as participants experience less anxiety than in large groups. Quinn (1995) identifies a variety of small learning groups such as 'snowball' groups, 'buzz' groups and 'crossover' groups.

Group work is best facilitated by encouraging participants to arrange themselves in a circle so that they can all see each other. They should be seated either on the floor (floor cushions are a kindness) or on chairs of equal height to ensure that they can see and hear each other, and to avoid any sense of inequalities. For subgroup work, the room needs to be large enough to accommodate several subgroups, or, alternatively, there needs to be access to smaller rooms nearby.

Within either large or small groups, other techniques can be used, such as brainstorming to generate ideas, and the use of flip-chart paper to write and display the generated ideas. It is important to note that, when using groups for any activity, the dynamics of that group play a part in the form that responses may take. Facilitators need to attend to the verbal and nonverbal communication of each member in the group, including their own. It is useful to recognize that, for every action in the group, be it verbal or nonverbal, there will be a reaction. It is part of the facilitator's role to monitor these reactions and, if necessary, guide them towards a constructive end.

Individual Work

The prime purpose of individual work is for personal reflection of what has been, or is being, learned. It can be used in conjunction with group work. An example of this occurs in the workshop in Chapter 5, where participants are encouraged to reflect upon particular issues in each section of the workshop. However, individual work can also be used to provide a time for reflections that are for each participant's sole use and do not have to be communicated to anyone unless they choose to do so. Similarly, evaluations offer a space for reflection on the workshop outcomes and may be shared with the group or retained by the individual.

Exercises

These are activities that can be structured or unstructured. They are usually short in duration and are used to help people to get to know each other; help them to begin to feel more relaxed at the start of a workshop; introduce a focal topic through a less intense experience; or help to maintain motivation during the workshop. They are also important in helping people to recognize the activity base for learning and that learning can be enjoyable and fun. Exercises can be identified as 'games' with a win–lose criterion, for example, the game 'Time Bomb' in Chapter 8. In this exercise the last person left in the group is the winner. Contrast this with the exercise in Chapter 6 called 'Rainstorm', which is there to help to increase a feeling of group cohesion and in which there is no winner. The amount of structure in exercises can be variable, ranging from the only instruction of one exercise being to 'build a structure with bodies' to the requirement that participants perform a sequence of tasks in a particular order (see Exercise 7.3: Shaking off the Dog).

It is important for facilitators to note that exercises must be genuinely offered with no-one being forced to participate, as this would be counter-motivational, potentially disrupting the whole group cohesion and the desire to learn. This caution is one that applies to all experiential learning activities. If participants are not fully co-operative, then a positive learning outcome is less likely. Having said this, reluctant participants should be strongly encouraged to meet their obligations to themselves and fellow learners, but their right of refusal to participate must always be respected, although they could be asked to provide insights into the learning process as an independent observer.

Structured Experiences

These are exercises that are generally of a longer duration and often have no associated win–lose criterion. They focus upon the main subject area within a particular workshop or part of the workshop. Pfeiffer and Jones' (1969–1985) series of handbooks offer excellent examples of structured experiences to explore specific areas. They often have a defined sequence of events, identifiable outcomes, and recognized roles for participants. The exercises can be undertaken in small or large groups, which may include all of the participants or small groupings. Invariably there is a plenary feedback session in which the whole group discusses the exercise and its meaning for their learning. In all experiential work, this reflection is vital to encourage productive learning. The caution about reluctant participants mentioned in the section on 'Exercises' also applies to structured experiences.

Additionally, there is value in either adapting structured experiences that do not completely meet the facilitator's or the group's requirements (this is especially important where the exercise was developed in one country and put to use in another, e.g. USA to UK) or developing experiences from scratch, which, although time consuming, will more precisely meet the needs of the workshop.

Role Play

This activity offers participants the opportunity to simulate a real event within a safe environment. Two or more individuals participate in the role play, which may be structured or unstructured. An example of a structured role play is given in Chapter 9, where both the health care worker and client are given specific roles and asked to act in a particular way. An unstructured role play is exemplified in Chapter 6, where only general instructions are given to the participants and they must create the specifics of that scene.

It is also possible to encourage participants to devise 'on the spot' scenarios, especially to deal with issues brought from the clinical setting, by asking questions such as: 'Would you like to use role play to work on something?', 'What would you like to work on?', 'What roles are involved?', 'How would you like the roles to be enacted?', 'Who would like to take a particular role?', etc. In this way, health care workers can gain an insight into different ways of managing communications with clients. Also, by using the technique of role reversal, it is possible to develop an insight into what it might be like to be in the client's position. The value of using role play in learning that is skills based and also has a high emotional content as in health care, is that the practitioner has an opportunity to experience both skills and emotions, and not just the cognitive aspect of care.

In conducting role play, facilitators need to attend to a number of issues. First, it is important that the role play is as realistic as possible. This can be achieved without vast outlay on props and equipment, by drawing upon the participants' own experiences. This will make the subject matter relevant to the participants and also relate it more closely to what they need to learn, especially the skills required for competent practice.

Secondly, facilitators should ensure that the role play scene is not interrupted by either the facilitator or the other participants, unless the technique of 'shadowing' or 'role replacement' has been agreed upon. Shadowing is a technique by which the action of the role play is momentarily frozen by all the players at the request of one of them, and nonparticipating observers are invited to 'speak for' one of the actors, usually by standing behind the person they will speak for, with a hand upon that person's shoulder. Role replacement is similar to this, with the exception that the actor steps aside and the replacement takes over the role completely. This can be of particular value in one to one interactions to give participants the opportunity to view the world from the other person's point of view.

Thirdly, it is very important that the participants are debriefed or de-roled (see Chapter 1 for a method of doing this). This brings participants out of the role they were in, together with its attendant thoughts, feelings and behaviours. Debriefing helps to 'ground' the person back in reality and may also help people to draw conclusions from the role play (van Ments, 1992).

Role play may be further enhanced when combined with video recording equipment. Reviews of studies comparing the effectiveness of role playing with and without video indicates that the use of video and audio equipment markedly increases the effectiveness of social skills training (Bailey and Sowder, 1970; Griffiths, 1974). However, the use of video can create anxiety among participants, especially when being used for the first time (Raymond et al. 1993). Nevertheless, where initial anxiety can be overcome, the use of video equipment can prove a valuable learning tool (Minardi and Riley, 1991).

Participants should be encouraged to use the video equipment. All of the equipment should be set up before it is needed so they can become accustomed to its presence. The operators of the equipment must be advised to record only material relevant to the role play and not to record peripheral activities. The equipment or any material recorded should not be used in a frivolous way, otherwise a potentially valuable learning tool may be trivialized and abused.

The advantage of having a video recording of the communications is that participants can view their actions and reactions, replaying as necessary to derive maximum information for reflection/discussion. Observing oneself 'on screen' also has the potential for learning even in the absence of others' comments. As well as hearing the verbal content, the participants are able to see more clearly their nonverbal responses, which are often out of awareness while the interaction is taking place. Video recordings offer other participants an opportunity to identify communication related issues that they may have missed first time around. Finally, it presents as an opportunity for vicarious learning.

Using these methods for communication skills training can enhance skills acquisition and extend the competence of practitioners. However, they are powerful tools and, if used incautiously, they have the potential to negate the learning experience. Facilitators should use these techniques with care, but above all with creativity and genuineness. This will result in a meaningful and productive learning experience.

Summary

This chapter has focused on how competent communication skills may be acquired by health care workers. It has also identified the complexities of developing an ability to recognize how, what, where, when and with whom it is necessary to communicate, identifying some of the innate aspects of language (Sutherland, 1992) as well as the extent to which it is environmentally driven.

The needs of adult learners have been considered and, in particular, the importance of this for health care workers. The use of experiential techniques has been advocated as a fruitful teaching strategy for adult learners and the main methods employed in the workshops have been described. These issues have been examined in relation to the acquisition of effective communication skills. This and other chapters in Part I of the book have presented a theoretical overview. What is now required to develop the actual skills in communicating effectively is an identification of the standards, practice and feedback on the use of these skills. This is the focus for Part II, which is designed to provide a variety of learning experiences, from a total communications curriculum to a single exercise in raising an awareness of one aspect of communication. Whichever way Part II is used, it is hoped that this chapter and the others in Part I have provided enough theory about communication and how it may be taught to enable the reader to utilize the second part with confidence and competence.

Communication Skills Workshops

Chapter 5

Communication Skills: an Overview

This introductory workshop forms the basis of work later to be explored in more depth. It is designed to give an overview of the basic components of communication, verbal and nonverbal, with active listening as the bridge between the two. It also begins the process of skills training in communication, introducing participants to the possibly unfamiliar world of experiential learning. Whether the workshop is used as the first of a sequence or as a single episode of training, we suggest that facilitators should pay particular attention to providing enough time to enable participants to overcome any anxieties. This entails proper preparation, perhaps by giving participants a copy of the learning outcomes prior to the workshop, and ensuring that there is enough time during the sessions for explanations, encouragement and a sense that the workshop can be fun rather than an ordeal.

We acknowledge that using and practising some of the techniques might feel awkward and artificial, whether to learn new skills or refresh old ones. Persuasion to overcome this (often transient) sense of embarrassment needs to come not only from facilitators but also from the participants themselves. We have found that one of the keys to running successful communications workshops is to encourage participants to offer feedback to each other. In doing this they are more able to overcome any sense of awkwardness in a possibly unfamiliar learning environment, and, moreover, will be able to share their own skills and knowledge to the benefit of their peers and ultimately their clients.

Learning Outcomes

1. Identify why communication skills are important in health care;
2. Recognize the difference between verbal and nonverbal skills;

3. Recognize the interdependence of verbal and nonverbal skills in effective communication;
4. Identify what is involved in active listening;
5. Practise the use and recognition of verbal, nonverbal and active listening skills;
6. Reflect upon significant reactions/feelings/thoughts experienced when using the above skills.

Introduction to the Workshop

The facilitators need to state:

- *Learning outcomes for the workshop*
- *Methods used* Spend some time discussing this and allaying anxieties at this initial workshop. Suggest that participation in the exercises will enhance learning and their enjoyment of the workshop, but let participants know that they will not be forced to take part in any exercise if they do not wish to do so.
- *Time considerations* Make explicit the overall time for the workshop, and the time taken for breaks and when these might occur. Negotiate some flexibility in timing (up to 15 minutes either side of a stated time) but ensure that you finish the day on time.
- *Housekeeping issues* Locations of other rooms, toilet facilities, and eating and drinking arrangements; rules about smoking (e.g. designated areas, although we advise not to allow smoking during the workshop); issues concerning participants' safety, including fire procedures and those relating to personal items such as clothing, jewellery and footwear.

Theory Input: Teaching Communications Skills

- *Outcomes*
  Recognize processes and methods of communication;
  Identify a rationale for teaching communications skills;
  Recognize the value of effective communication with clients/patients.
- *Configuration*
  The whole group.
- *Time*
  Approximately 20 minutes.

● *Materials*
None.

● *Process*
All humans are in continuous communication with each other, either through verbal or nonverbal means. When verbally transmitting messages, there is a need to communicate clearly in order for this message to be received as accurately as possible. Nonverbal messages are transmitted through a variety of means such as prosodics (rhythm, pauses, intonation), facial expression, gestures and other behaviours, paralanguage, and standing features (i.e. appearance related to clothes, hair style, etc.) (Ellis and Beattie, 1986). Therefore, it is necessary to attend to all of the verbal and nonverbal messages that you send and receive. Also, because interpersonal communication is a two-way process, it is important to attend to the total communication (i.e. verbal and nonverbal) from the client.

It is interesting to note that various aspects of communication are learned at a very early age. Sutherland (1992) proposed that infants up to three months of age can imitate the vocal sounds and gestures of adults. Eimas *et al.* (1971) have suggested that a one-month-old child is able to discriminate differences between two sounds, implying that processing and internalization of communication takes place very early in human development. This suggests that communication ability forms first at a nonverbal level and subsequently develops verbally, enabling messages to be sent and received as accurately as possible. During development, children learn to 'decentre' or become less self-centred in their communication, until as adults they can understand and communicate taking into account another person's viewpoint (Donaldson, 1978). Within this perspective, it is necessary to recognize the influence of environmental and personal contexts on the communication being transmitted and received. Therefore, the level of decentring and the recognition of these contexts by the sender and the recipient will affect how communications are transmitted and/or received.

It is essential to be aware of the tendency for people to develop idiosyncratic patterns of communication when relaying some messages (e.g. those that help to make emotional distress palatable or those that produce an unconscious response). Generally, this learned pattern is effective in transmitting or receiving the correct messages. However, at times, the desired message is not received or sent as intended. This may be the result of a number of factors, one of which is that the patterns of communication used previously are inappropriate in the present context. In order to alter this situation, it becomes necessary to bring unconscious patterns into consciousness so they can be altered, resulting in more effective communication.

The difference between the conscious and unconscious use of communication in health care settings is succinctly described by Macleod Clark (1981). By teaching communication skills, an attempt is being made to raise communication awareness from an unconscious to a conscious level. This serves two purposes. First, it enables carers to recognize and alter faulty communication patterns and secondly it enables an increase in the conscious repertoire of skills available for use by health care workers with clients. Although it is likely that these skills will become unconscious again, their retrieval will be more rapid and a larger variety of skills will be available to use in different situations.

An overall model of communication is presented by Ellis and Beattie (1986) (see Chapter 2, Figure 2.2). However, the model used for examining communication skills in this and subsequent workshops is:

- Verbal communication;
- Nonverbal communication;
- Active listening.

Verbal communications can be identified as those that involve speech (though Argyle (1988) has also placed writing and sign within this domain) and its component parts (e.g. words, clauses, sentences) (Ellis and Beattie, 1986). It serves a number of purposes, some of which are to exchange information, clarify issues, demonstrate understanding, and offer support and/or direction.

Nonverbal communication is understood to be all other modes of communication not in the verbal arena. Thus facial expression, gesture, body posture, gaze, distance, appearance, paralinguistics, silence, etc. would come into this category. A number of the nonverbal communications listed can be further subdivided. For example, Argyle (1983) differentiates gaze and eye contact. He suggests that eye contact relates to a high level of pupil to pupil contact such as in intimate relationships and superordinate/subordinate relationships, while gaze consists of generally looking at the other person's face, occasionally looking at their eyes, and also at times looking away from the face. It has also been identified that vocalizations such as 'umm' and 'ah' are considered part of the paralinguistic system and therefore are nonverbal (Argyle, 1983; Ellis and Beattie, 1986; Porritt, 1990; Trower et al. 1978). Argyle (1988) has suggested that nonverbal communication serves five purposes: (1) expressing emotion; (2) communicating interpersonal attitudes; (3) accompanying and supporting speech; (4) self presentation; and (5) rituals. With such a large role in communication, it is not surprising that Birdwhistell (1970) found that 65% of all human communication is nonverbal.

Active listening in these workshops is seen as the bridge between verbal and nonverbal communication. This is because it uses both forms of communication (see Chapter 2, Figure 2.3). That is, when actively listening, you are not only listening to various aspects of the person's speech, but also observing the nonverbal messages being expressed. However, active listening does not just focus upon the client, because it is necessary to monitor – or 'actively listen' – to your own verbal and nonverbal communication and alter this if it seems necessary or is feasible. One model of active listening used in this and subsequent workshops is that of Watts (1986), which consists of: (1) listening to the manifest content; (2) reading between the lines; and (3) listening to the latent content of the client's speech (see Chapter 8 for a more comprehensive description). Active listening, therefore, not only identifies listening to the client attentively but also demonstrates to the client that you are listening by clarifying, checking your understanding and theirs, recognizing and responding to cues from the latent content of their speech, and feeding that back to them where appropriate.

It is crucial to recognize the importance of communication techniques that may improve the effectiveness of health care workers being able to identify the types of messages – verbal or nonverbal – that may be transmitted from the client and/or to the client. By becoming conscious of communication patterns that have been learned over the years, we are more likely to use communication appropriate to the situation and the client. This will result in being able to help them to retain their dignity and as much independence as possible, regardless of the circumstances they are experiencing.

Exercise 5.1: Brainstorm – Components of Communication

● *Outcomes*
Begin the process of consciously considering the types of communications used;
Make a conscious separation of verbal from nonverbal communication;
Identify the amount of discrete verbal and nonverbal communication in our messages;
Identify the difficulty in separating the verbal and nonverbal components of communication in our messages.

- *Configuration*
  The whole group.
- *Time*
  Twenty minutes.
- *Materials*
  Flip-chart paper, chalk board or white board;
  Appropriate writing implements;
  Blu-tac.
- *Process*
  Use six large pieces of paper tacked together on the wall (or white board/chalk board) to write down the items of the brainstorm. Ask all students to identify verbal and nonverbal components of communication, writing their own contributions on the paper or white board.
  Do not isolate items of the brainstorm until after it is finished.
  Facilitator(s) may wish to contribute other types of communication that have not been mentioned by the students.
  Ask the students to identify the items in the respective components of verbal (responding and questioning) and nonverbal communication, and a student or tutor to circle each in a different coloured pen (one colour for verbal and another for nonverbal). It is important to have identified in the brainstorm that paralinguistics (e.g. the 'mmms' and 'hmms' of speech) are classified as nonverbal communications. If this comes up as a controversy, it can be productive to encourage discussion, as it often results in a creative exploration of views, suggesting that these vocal aspects of communication do not contain words and hence are not considered verbal communication.
  Examples of some verbal and nonverbal communications are:
  Verbal Open questions, clarifying questions, probing questions, reflection, echoing, paraphrasing, open statements, summarizing, closed questions (occasionally considered skilled), multiple questions (not usually considered skilled).
  Nonverbal Nods of the head, facial expression, body posture, gestures, eye gaze, eye contact, body contact, personal space, paralinguistics, voice pitch/tone/speed, appearance, smells, silence.

Introduction to Verbal Communication Skills

Exercise 5.2: Warm Up – Fists

- *Outcomes*
  Begin the process of focusing upon verbal communication;
  Fun.

- *Configuration*
  Pairs.
- *Time*
  Five minutes.
- *Materials*
  None.
- *Process*
  Participants must use verbal communication only, no physical contact is allowed.
  Participants break into pairs.
  One person identifies herself or himself as 'A' and the other as 'B'.
  'B' clenches her or his hand into a fist and 'A' tries to persuade her/him to unclench it. The person clenching the fist should only do so if persuaded to by his or her partner.
  After two minutes, the individuals in each pair reverse roles.

Exercise 5.3: Chinese Whispers

- *Outcomes*
  Experience how verbal messages can be distorted during transmission;
  Demonstrate the importance of listening very carefully in the absence of nonverbal signals;
  Fun.
- *Configuration*
  The whole group.
- *Time*
  Five minutes.
- *Materials*
  A prepared message.
- *Process*
  The group stands or sits in a circle so that each person is about two feet away from all the others.
  One of the group facilitators whispers the following message to the person on his or her right, so no-one else can hear: 'The next train for Manchester will be leaving from platform four in 20 minutes. It is the last train today.'
  The statement is said *once* only in a clear, slow voice; it must *not* be repeated.
  That person then passes the message on to the person on his or her right, again in a whisper, not repeated, and so no-one else will hear.

This same procedure is followed until everyone in the group has been passed the message.

The last person to receive the message says it aloud. It is checked with the original statement for accuracy perhaps using a previously prepared overhead projector transparency or by writing the message up for all to see.

Exercise 5.4: Questioning and Responding

- *Outcomes*
  Practise making conscious use of the questioning and responding skills identified in the previous brainstorm (Exercise 5.1);
  Practise offering constructive feedback to each other in relation to the skills used;
  Help to build cohesiveness in the group.

- *Configuration*
  Pairs.

- *Time*
  Total: 20 minutes (approximately five minutes per person in each role and 10 minutes for the small group feedback/discussion session).

- *Materials*
  None.

- *Process*
  One person is identified as 'A' and the other as 'B' (encourage participants to work with a different person from previous exercises).

  'A' questions 'B' about how this person spent the three weeks prior to starting this course or work, and 'B' responds to 'A' appropriately.

  Reverse roles so that 'B' is the questioner and 'A' the responder. Both 'A' and 'B' should attempt to use the verbal communications discussed in the introduction and brainstorm session.

  It is important to tell the pairs that *both participants* may use questioning and responding skills in each of the sessions, but that the person designated as questioner or responder will focus mainly on either questioning or responding as appropriate to their assigned role.

  Ask participants to feedback in small groups of four or six, to discuss the following:
    Were they able to use forms of questions?
    What did it feel like to ask/receive these forms of questions?

Were they able to use different forms of responses?
What did it feel like to give/receive different forms of responses?
What helped/hindered the communication to develop/continue?

Exercise 5.5: 'Turn-Taking'

● *Outcomes*
Experience a verbal interaction when the participants do not take turns;
Experience a verbal interaction when participants take turns as normal in that conversation;
Develop group cohesiveness.

● *Configuration*
Pairs.

● *Time*
Total: five minutes (approximately one minute for Part 1 and two minutes for Part 2).

● *Materials*
None.

● *Process*
Identify this as an element of verbal communication (i.e. for effective communication, turn-taking must take place).
One person is identified as 'A' and the other as 'B' (encourage participants to work with a different person than in the previous exercises).
This exercise is in two parts:
　　(1) A and B talk about their previous day's events at same time.
　　(2) A and B talk about the previous day's events, taking turns as in normal conversation.
Concentrate only on the overt content of the speech and the verbal techniques used in turn-taking.

Plenary Discussion of Exercises 5.4 and 5.5

● *Outcomes*
Share thoughts and feelings in relation to the experience of conversations when 'turn-taking' is not involved and when it is involved.
Share thoughts and feelings about practising the conscious use of questioning and responding.
Share thoughts and feelings about the effect that nonverbal cues have on passing verbal messages accurately.

- *Configuration*
  The whole group.
- *Time*
  Approximately 30 minutes.
- *Process*
  Discuss the turn-taking exercise using the following questions:
  What did it feel like to talk at your partner and be talked *at* by your partner?
  What did it feel like talking with your partner?
  What helped/hindered you when taking turns?
  What verbal techniques were you able to identify in turn-taking?
  Discuss participants' thoughts and feelings about Exercises 5.4 and 5.5.
  Discuss whether or not they were able to try verbal communication techniques that were new.
  Discuss what thoughts and feelings were experienced when using verbal communication skills at a conscious level.

Exercise 5.6: Individual Reflection – Verbal Communication

- *Outcomes*
  Assist the participants to reflect upon what has just been experienced;
  Help participants to organize their thoughts about the session on verbal communication;
  Help the participants' recall when evaluating the day.
- *Configuration*
  The whole group as individuals.
- *Time*
  Fifteen minutes.
- *Materials*
  Individual reflection sheets (Figure 5.1).
- *Process*
  Using the individual reflection sheet (Figure 5.1), write and/or draw any thoughts the participant may have about the session on verbal communication.
  The facilitator states that what is recorded is solely for the participant's use and encourages participants to use these reflections at a later stage to further their own studies.

Use this sheet to write and/or sketch any significant reactions/feeling/thoughts you have experienced in each of the following sessions of the day. This sheet is for your use only and does NOT have to be shared with anyone.

You may wish to use your personal reflections at some later stage to guide your own further reading on the subject of communication skills.

Verbal communication session:

Nonverbal communication session:

Active listening session:

Figure 5.1 Individual reflections

Introduction to Nonverbal Communication Skills

Facilitators should discuss the nonverbal element of communication, reiterating Birdwhistell's (1970) suggestion that 65% of human communication is nonverbal. Propose that, while individuals rely on verbal cues in interactions, nonverbal cues (gestures, posture, tone of voice, etc.) are important in order for communications to be effective. Remind participants that incongruence between verbal and nonverbal messages can be confusing for the recipient and possibly cause psychological distress. Ask participants for examples of incongruent verbal/nonverbal messages, or, using a volunteer, the facilitator states to the volunteer, 'I like you', but using an angry tone of voice and an angry facial expression and gestures. Lead a brief discussion asking participants what needed to be different to give the message 'I like you' its full, genuine meaning.

Exercise 5.7: Warm Up – Mirror

- *Outcomes*
  Help participants to become more aware of nonverbal messages; Fun.
- *Configuration*
  Pairs.
- *Time*
  Ten minutes.
- *Materials*
  None.
- *Process*
  The group divides into pairs, designating each other as 'A' or 'B' (encourage participants to work with different people in this whole section).
  'A' plays the part of a mirror and 'B' the individual standing in front of the mirror.
  'B' then moves in whatever way is desired and 'A' must mimic 'B' in the same way that a mirror does (e.g. if 'B' raises his or her *right* arm, then, as a mirror image, 'A' moves his or her *left* arm.
  Emphasize that no verbal communication must be used.
  After five minutes, 'A' and 'B' reverse roles and repeat the process.

Exercise 5.8: Nonverbal Signals – Position

- *Outcomes*
  Experience the way in which body orientation (proxemics) plays a part in communication;
  Discuss the impact of body position on communication and the feelings of being both the giver and the recipient of a communication in those circumstances.
- *Configuration*
  Pairs and small groups of four or six.
- *Time*
  15 minutes (approximately three minutes per position and five minutes for small group discussion).
- *Materials*
  None.
- *Process*
  The group divides into pairs (participants preferably pairing with people with whom they have not yet worked).

The pairs first sit *back to back* and talk about any subject they choose for approximately three minutes.

After the time is up, they sit *side by side* (directly side by side) and continue the conversation from the first part of the exercise for a further three minutes.

The participants then sit *facing* each other in as comfortable a way as possible and again, for three minutes, carry on the conversation that took place in the previous two sections of the exercise.

After the three parts of the exercise are finished, each pair joins with one or two other pairs (the group should preferably be no larger than four or six participants). They discuss the impact of position upon their ability to communicate with each other, focusing on what particularly helped or hindered the flow of the conversation.

Exercise 5.9: Nonverbal Signals – Distance/Personal Space

- *Outcomes*
  Experience holding a conversation in which the participants are at different distances from each other;
  Experience and identify the feelings associated with being at these distances.

- *Configuration*
  Pairs and small groups of four to six.

- *Time*
  Total: 15 minutes.

- *Materials*
  Ruler.

- *Process*
  Remind participants that incongruence between verbal and non-verbal messages can at the least cause some confusion in the message that recipients receive, and, at worst, it can cause severe psychological distress in the recipient.
  Suggest that, while individuals rely on verbal cues in interactions, nonverbal cues (gestures, posture, tone of voice, etc.) are important in order for communications to be effective.
  Exemplify the importance of nonverbal messages and how they can change the meaning of a communication.
  The group divides into pairs.
  Pairs first communicate with each other from opposite sides of the room, talking for three minutes about any subject they choose.
  After the time is up, they communicate with each other while six

inches apart (using a ruler placed nose to nose to measure the distance), continuing the conversation from the first part of the exercise for a further three minutes (the facilitator may frequently need to encourage the pairs to maintain a six-inch distance from each other!).

After three minutes, the participants communicate with each other from a distance at which they feel comfortable and again for three minutes carry on the conversation that took place in the previous two sections of the exercise.

When all three parts of the exercise are complete, the pairs join together to make small groups (no more than six participants per group) to discuss the impact of distance upon their ability to communicate, focusing upon what helped and what hindered the progress of the communication.

Exercise 5.10: Nonverbal Signals – Eye Contact/Gaze

- *Outcomes*
  Experience holding a conversation when eye contact/gaze is being used in three different ways;
  Experience and identify the feelings associated with differing levels of gaze/eye contact.

- *Configuration*
  Pairs and small groups of four to six participants.

- *Time*
  Total: 15 minutes.

- *Materials*
  None.

- *Process*
  The group divides into pairs and identify each other as 'A' or 'B'.
  While talking for about three minutes about any subject they wish, 'A' looks 'B' in the eyes while 'B' looks down or away.
  After the time is up, 'B' looks 'A' in the eyes while 'A' looks down or away and they continue the conversation from the first part of the exercise for a further three minutes.
  'A' and 'B' then look at each other in what they consider to be a normal way and again carry on the conversation that took place in the previous two sections of the exercise for a further three minutes.

Plenary Discussion of Exercises 5.8, 5.9 and 5.10

- *Outcomes*
  Explore how body position, distance and eye contact/gaze can influence the flow of an interaction;
  Differentiate eye contact from gaze (see 'Theory Input');
  Explore, in general, how nonverbal communication can effect an interaction.
- *Configuration*
  The whole group.
- *Time*
  Approximately 20 minutes.
- *Process*
  Have the whole group sitting close to each other (e.g. in a circle), either on chairs, the floor or cushions, etc.
  Discuss what it felt like to be interacting when eye contact and gaze were/were not made (restating the distinction between eye contact and gaze), in different positions and at different distances.
  Discuss what may have helped and/or hindered the flow of communication in the exercises.
  Widen the discussion to the effect that nonverbal communication may have on any interaction and ask for any further considerations about Birdwhistell's (1970) assertion that about 65% of all of our face to face communications are nonverbal.

Exercise 5.11: Individual Reflection – Nonverbal Communication

- *Outcomes*
  Assist the participants to reflect upon what has just been experienced;
  Help participants to organize their thoughts about the session on nonverbal communication;
  Help the participants' recall when evaluating the day.
- *Configuration*
  The whole group as individuals.
- *Time*
  Fifteen minutes.
- *Materials*
  Individual reflection sheets (Figure 5.1).
- *Process*
  Using an individual reflection sheet (Figure 5.1), each participant

writes and/or draws any thoughts he or she may have about the session on nonverbal communication.
The facilitator states that what is recorded is solely for the participant's use

Theory Input: Introduction to Active Listening

- *Outcomes*
  Differentiate active from passive listening;
  Relate active listening to verbal and nonverbal communications;
  Identify that active listening relates to hidden/unconscious messages in a client's speech, with the listener attempting to clarify and facilitate the client to put meaning into these messages.
- *Configuration*
  The whole group.
- *Time*
  Approximately 15 minutes.
- *Materials*
  None.
- *Process*
  Listening is not only done with your ears but with other senses, such as vision, smell, and touch. Using all of our senses makes it possible to pick up the whole message from clients. Thus an important function of active listening is to increase awareness of clients' nonverbal messages and identify whether or not they are congruent with the verbal ones (e.g. they say everything is OK, while shaking their heads, giving the signal 'No'). Active listening combines verbal and nonverbal communication, helping the health care worker to focus upon the overt and the latent (i.e. hidden/unconscious) content of the client's speech. This involves listening intently to the client's verbal and nonverbal messages, and responding appropriately to these. In contrast, passive listening only uses the aural channel and does not include responding to the client as does active listening.

  It is important to be alert to times when the client speaks very softly, mumbles, or invents words, as this could signal difficult or important issues for the client. Attention to such detail can help to identify unpalatable material, which is often spoken just prior to or during their inaudible or distorted verbalizations. In this instance, by using verbal communication to clarify what the speaker is saying, you are also informing her or him that you have understood (or are trying to understand) the communication.

This will help the client to feel valued and demonstrates that they have been listened to empathically. It may be possible that the concern raised by this communication is one not in the client's conscious awareness. The health care worker needs to recognize this form of communication and respond by identifying the issue at an appropriate moment in the interaction. It is useful for carers to recognize – and consider the purpose of – times when a client is not allowing the usual flow of conversation (i.e. not always allowing 'turn-taking').

In active listening, it is crucial for health care workers to attend to their own verbal and nonverbal messages as well as those of the client. In responding verbally, they need consciously to choose the words used and be aware of the nonverbal signals they are transmitting. This will help to ensure that the nonverbal messages are congruent with the verbal messages and that the verbal messages are relevant to the verbal and/or nonverbal ones from the client. Active listening, therefore, means that you take an *active* part in what is being expressed by the client. You need to listen to the actual content of the client's speech, attempting to understand word meanings (as well as 'listening' to nonverbal signals), the context within which the client is speaking, and the context (either overt or covert) that surrounds what is being said by the client. With this information, you need to be an active participant in the interaction, through verbally clarifying and summarizing, and nonverbally demonstrating your presence for the client. It is this aspect of communication (i.e. active listening) that the remainder of the workshop will address.

Exercise 5.12: Warm Up – Story Circle

- *Outcomes*
  Help the participants to focus upon accurate listening;
  Identify what it feels like to listen and speak to someone without seeing them;
  Use of imagination;
  Fun.
- *Configuration*
  The whole group.
- *Time*
  Approximately five minutes, times the number of participants in the group.
- *Materials*
  None.

● *Process*
Participants lie on their backs in a circle on the floor with their heads towards the centre. Alternatively, they can sit on chairs in a circle with their backs to the centre.

The facilitator then instructs them that he or she will start a story and, after two minutes, will tap a participant's foot once.

That participant must continue the story until his or her foot is tapped twice by the facilitator.

The facilitator will then tap another participant's foot once and the story line will shift to that person until his or her foot is tapped twice.

This process will continue until all have had an opportunity to participate in telling the story.

It is important to reiterate at the beginning of the warm up that the story line is continuous throughout the exercise.

Exercise 5.13: Listening Actively

● *Outcomes*
Experience listening actively to another person and being actively listened to at a conscious level;

Recognize the feelings and thoughts associated with being an active listener and being actively listened to;

Identify the components of being an active listener;

Explore thoughts and feelings associated with being actively listened to and listening actively to another person.

● *Configuration*
Pairs.

● *Time*
Total: 15 minutes (approximately five minutes for each person taking the listener role and five minutes for a small discussion after both participants have been the active listener).

● *Materials*
None.

● *Process*
The group divides into pairs and each person identifies as 'A' or 'B'.

'A' then talks with 'B' about any subject (e.g. 'winter') for five minutes and 'B' listens *actively*.

After the time is up, they reverse roles so that 'B' speaks for five minutes and 'A' listens actively.

When the time is up, both participants discuss the thoughts and feelings associated with listening and being listened to actively, in terms of what helped or hindered the conversation and what components of active listening they could identify.

Exercise 5.14: Not Listening Actively

- *Outcomes*
  Experience actively not listening to another person and not being actively listened to at a conscious level;
  Recognize the feelings and thoughts associated with not listening and not being actively listened to;
  Explore thoughts and feelings associated with actively not being listened to and not listening actively to another person.
- *Configuration*
  Pairs.
- *Time*
  Total: 10 minutes (approximately five minutes for each person taking the nonlistener role).
- *Materials*
  None.
- *Process*
  The group remains in the same pairs as the last exercise.
  Each person in the pair again identifies who is 'A' and who is 'B'.
  'A' then talks with 'B' about any subject, (e.g. 'summer', for five minutes) and 'B' actively does not listen to 'A' (i.e. does not attend to 'A') and makes responses/asks questions that are incongruent to 'A''s material.
  After the time is up, they reverse roles so that 'B' speaks for five minutes and 'A' actively does not listen to 'B'.

Plenary Discussion of Exercises 5.13 and 5.14

- *Outcomes*
  Share thoughts and feelings about not being actively listened to and having not actively listened to someone else;
  Discuss the use of active listening in developing and maintaining an effective client–practitioner relationship.
- *Configuration*
  The whole group.
- *Time*
  Approximately 15 minutes.

- *Process*
  The whole group sits close to each other (e.g. in a circle, either on chairs, the floor, cushions, etc.).
  Discuss thoughts and feelings about the last two exercises in the group that were associated with being the listener/nonlistener and being listened to/not listened to, in terms of what helped or hindered the conversation.
  Open up to a general discussion about active listening and what might help or hinder effective interactions between the practitioner and client.

Exercise 5.15: Individual Reflection – Active Listening

- *Outcomes*
  Assist the participants to reflect upon what has just been experienced;
  Help participants to organize their thoughts about the session on active listening;
  Help participants to recall when evaluating the day.
- *Configuration*
  The whole group as individuals.
- *Time*
  Fifteen minutes.
- *Materials*
  Individual reflection sheets (Figure 5.1).
- *Process*
  Using the individual reflection sheet (Figure 5.1), the participant writes and/or draws any thoughts he or she may have about the session on active listening.
  The facilitator states that what is recorded is solely for the participant's use.

Exercise 5.16: Evaluation of the Workshop

- *Outcomes*
  Help the participants to identify what they liked most and what they liked least about the workshop;
  Help the facilitator(s) to identify what parts of the workshop were liked and what parts might need alteration;
  Offer the participants practice in giving negative and positive feedback.
- *Configuration*
  The whole group.

- *Time*
  Approximately 15 minutes.
- *Materials*
  None.
- *Process*
  The participants sit on chairs in a circle.
  Ask each member to say one thing they liked least about the whole workshop or 'pass'; they are requested not to respond to any request for justification of their statement.
  After each has done this, ask them to say one thing they liked most about the whole workshop or 'pass'; they are requested not to give or respond to any request for justification of their statement.
  The facilitator(s) of the workshop must also be included.

Exercise 5.17: End Game – Gift in a Shoe

- *Outcomes*
  Help participants to leave the workshop with positive feelings/thoughts about themselves;
  Enable people to respond only positively towards other workshop participants and the facilitators;
  Lighten the atmosphere of an intense workshop.
- *Configuration*
  The whole group.
- *Time*
  Approximately 20–30 minutes.
- *Materials*
  Small pieces of blank paper and pencils.
- *Process*
  Each group member is given small pieces of paper equal in number minus one (i.e. the one for themselves) to the participants, including the facilitators.
  Participants are each then asked to remove a shoe and place it in front of them to act as the receptacle for their 'gift'.
  On each piece of paper they write an individual's name and underneath, write and/or draw, something positive (it is important to make it explicit to participants that only positive comments are acceptable) about that person (e.g. their warmth, friendliness, nice clothes, pleasant voice, etc.).
  They may sign the slips of paper if they wish.
  Each participant deposits the slips of paper in the appropriate shoes, this being done either as they write/draw on each paper,

or at the end after they have written/drawn on all of the slips of paper.

After they have privately read them, the recipients of the 'gifts' may read any of them to the other participants.

The facilitator(s) then close the workshop.

Reading List

Argyle, M. (1988) *Bodily Communication*, 2nd ed. Routledge, London.

Ellis, A. and Beattie, G. (1986) *The Psychology of Language and Communication*. Lawrence Erlbaum, Hove.

Hargie, O., ed. (1986) *A Handbook of Communication Skills*. Routledge, London.

Porritt, L. (1990) *Interaction Strategies*, 2nd ed. Churchill Livingstone, Melbourne.

Chapter 6

Further Elements of Nonverbal Communication

In the process of communication, the nonverbal component is crucial. Arguably, this is the most ancient set of signals used by man, and remains, in general, the only form of communication used by animals other than humans (Pearce, 1987). Argyle (1988) has suggested that the functions of nonverbal communication are to communicate interpersonal attitudes and emotions, to present aspects of self, to enact rituals, and to support and enhance verbal communication. Until recently, health care workers have tended to focus primarily upon verbal communication, but there is increasing recognition of the importance of the nonverbal, such as the use of space or proxemics (Scheflen and Ashcraft, 1976) and the body or parts of the body (i.e. kinesics) (Birdwhistell, 1970; Pasquali *et al.* 1989).

This workshop builds upon that in Chapter 5, examining further aspects of nonverbal communication. Its structured exercises give the participants an opportunity to examine and discuss how their own nonverbal behaviours assist in communicating. It also offers an opportunity to explore the relationship between nonverbal communication and emotions. The value of recognizing this link is that it may be the only indication given of distress or pleasure by a client.

The first part of the workshop recommends the use of video cameras to record a role play. Some participants may find this difficult if they have not experienced this method of teaching and learning. It might be necessary to spend some time, either before the workshop or during the early part of it, in allowing them to express any anxieties. Similarly, feedback from the exercise might require allotted time to air reactions to this learning technique. It is also worth having the equipment already set up and available for inspection and use by participants to help to allay the anxiety of any participant who has not used video equipment before.

Learning Outcomes

1. Demonstrate knowledge of the components of nonverbal communication;
2. Explore how nonverbal communication may be presented and its effect on the interaction;
3. Share thoughts and feelings about the use of nonverbal communication;
4. Identify components of nonverbal communication and the emotions with which they may be associated;
5. Recognize the relationship between nonverbal communication and emotion;
6. Share thoughts and feelings about assumptions made between nonverbal communication and emotions.

Introduction to the Workshop

The facilitators need to state:

- *Learning outcomes for the workshop*
- *Methods used* Spend some time discussing this. Suggest that participation in the exercises will enhance learning and their enjoyment of the workshop, but let participants know that they will not be forced to take part if they do not wish to do so.
- *Time considerations* Make explicit the overall time for the workshop, and the time taken for breaks and when these might occur. Negotiate some flexibility in timing (up to 15 minutes either side of a stated time) but ensure that you finish on time.
- *Housekeeping issues* Locations of other rooms, toilet facilities, and eating and drinking arrangements; rules about smoking (e.g. designated areas, although we advise not to allow smoking during the workshop); issues concerning participants' safety, including fire procedures and those relating to personal items such as clothing, jewellery and footwear.

Exercise 6.1: Brainstorm – Components of Nonverbal Communication

- *Outcomes*
  Enable participants to recall and record elements of nonverbal communication;

Make a resource list of nonverbal elements of communication available for reference during the workshop.

- *Configuration*
  The whole group.
- *Time*
  Ten minutes.
- *Materials*
  Flip-chart paper, chalk board or white board;
  Appropriate writing implement;
  Blu-tac.
- *Process*
  The facilitator invites a volunteer to act as 'scribe' to the group.
  Individuals in the group (including the scribe) are asked to identify components of nonverbal communication.
  The scribe writes all the contributions on the flip-chart paper or board.
  If appropriate, the facilitator(s) add any relevant items not already identified.
  The completed list is pinned to the wall (or not erased from the board) for future reference during the remainder of the workshop.

Exercise 6.2: Warm Up – Rainstorm

- *Outcomes*
  Begin the process of group cohesion;
  Enable individuals to begin to feel comfortable with participation in workshop activities;
  Have fun.
- *Configuration*
  The whole group.
- *Time*
  Ten minutes.
- *Materials*
  None.
- *Process*
  The group sits in a circle with the facilitator standing in the middle.
  The facilitator then tells the group the sequence of events he or she would like them to perform, which is as follows:
  Clap hands;
  Slap both knees simultaneously;
  Slap both knees and stamp both feet simultaneously;

Slap both knees simultaneously;
Clap hands;
Stop all action.

The facilitator then tells the group that he or she will point to each participant in turn to indicate that group members should then clap their hands, continuing to do so until the facilitator next points to them.

After the whole group is clapping their hands, the facilitator points to each member in turn, at which time they should start slapping both knees simultaneously (remember that group members continue to clap their hands until pointed at to change behaviour to knee slapping).

After the whole group has begun to slap their knees, the facilitator again points to each in turn and they begin to slap their knees *and* stamp their feet on the floor (again group members must continue to slap their knees until pointed at to incorporate stamping their feet).

Next, the facilitator points to each person in turn just to slap their knees.

After each person is doing this, the facilitator points to each in turn to only clap their hands.

The final event is that the facilitator points to each group member in turn to stop all activity until the whole group is silent.

NB: The signalling to commence and cease activities is always done nonverbally (i.e. by pointing). It can be helpful for facilitators to demonstrate the sequence of activities to group members.

Exercise 6.3a: Role Play

- *Outcomes*
  Enable participants to identify the nonverbal communications used in 'everyday' situations;
  Encourage participants to explore how nonverbal communication may affect a conversation;
  Introduce participants to role playing as a learning method;
  Enable participants to become familiar with the use of a video camera as a learning tool in interpersonal skills training.

- *Configuration*
  The whole group.

- *Time*
  Approximately 35 minutes, consisting of 10 minutes for the introduction, 10 to 15 minutes to devise the role play, and 10 minutes to enact the scene.

- *Materials*
  A large room with chairs and tables;
  A supply of cups, jugs and bottles;
  Drinks (either plain water or a selection of soft drinks, if resources permit);
  A selection of snack foods (e.g. crisps and peanuts, if resources permit);
  Video camera, video recorder; television monitor (set up prior to the start of the workshop);
  Role play scenario: You are asked to play a scene in a pub. Six or seven people are already there. These people may be individuals or small groups of friends. The rest of the group comes into the pub (in groups or as individuals) and interact in whatever way they wish.
    You have 15 minutes in which to prepare. You therefore need to decide fairly quickly how you are going to organize the scene using the available 'props' in the room. You must also decide upon group and individual roles and have at least a rough idea about how different groups will interact with each other.
    The scene to be enacted will take no more than 10 minutes.
- *Process*
  The facilitator initially leads a discussion in which the role play set out above is introduced. The outcomes are made explicit and time is given to discussing the method (i.e. the use of video recordings). Participants are encouraged to express any concerns they may have about the use of video recording and their role in it.
  A copy of the role play scenario is given to the group.
  The members of the group are allowed up to 15 minutes to prepare their roles. (Try to avoid going over this time limit, as too much preparation time affects the impromptu nature of the scene and reduces the opportunity for spontaneous communication.)
  Participants are encouraged to use any items in the room as props and the facilitators help by providing any other items they can.
  After no more than 15 minutes, the participants enact the scene. This should be for approximately 10 minutes.
  The scene is then filmed either by the facilitators or one of the nonacting participants. The camera operator should use wide angle shots with slow sweeps across the scene, stopping to zoom in on and record scenes or interactions that show particular examples of nonverbal communication.
  At the end of 10 minutes, the facilitator calls the role play to a close.

NB: Participants should not be dragooned into this exercise. However, individuals who strongly object to participating in the role play should be encouraged to take part in other ways, such as taking on observer or technical roles (e.g. camera operator).

Exercise 6.3b: Alternative Role Play

- *Outcomes*

  Enable participants to identify the nonverbal communications used in 'everyday' situations;

  Allow participants to explore how nonverbal communication may affect a conversation;

  Introduce participants to role playing as a learning method.

- *Configuration*

  Small groups of between three and five participants.

- *Time*

  Approximately 25–35 minutes; five minutes for each scene and 10 minutes for feedback from the rest of the small group.

- *Materials*

  Role play scenarios (Table 6.1);

  Paper and pens.

- *Process*

  Within each small group, every member chooses one scene from Table 6.1.

  Each participant partners a person within the group. One of each pair becomes the observer.

  Each participant in turn enacts a chosen scene, using verbal and nonverbal communication. The participant enacting the scene may use other members of the group, but not the observer, as part of the role play. Members of the group not involved in the role play may wish to help the observer.

  The observer's role is to identify as many as possible nonverbal messages in the scene. Observations are written down for feedback later.

  After each scene, the observer leads a discussion about the scene. The observer and other group members offer feedback on nonverbal messages observed for about 10 minutes.

  This process continues until everyone in the small group has had a chance to act a scene and be an observer.

Table 6.1 Role play scenarios using nonverbal communication only

---

1. Find out whether or not your friend(s) in the cafeteria queue would like sugar in their coffee/tea and, if so, how much.

2. You have just dropped a tray full of cups and saucers. A terrible noise! You are lost for words. You apologize.

3. You are at a meeting and wish to be excused but do not want to disturb the others. Indicate your desire to the chairperson.

4. Your friend has indicated that he or she would like to leave the party. You do not want to leave. Tell him or her this.

5. You are in a meeting and you begin to feel sick. Indicate this to the person next to you and apologize to the speaker as you rush out.

6. You want to make some notes. You do not have a pen. Ask for one from some classmates.

7. You are at a party and think it is time to go home. Indicate this to a friend across the room.

8. You are getting a cold. You try to hold back your sneezes but you have not got a tissue. Indicate this.

9. Your friend is a bit drunk and feeling generous. He or she is about to lend £30.00 to a stranger. Attract his or her attention and indicate to him or her not to do this.

10. The sun suddenly begins to shine right into your eyes. You would like someone to draw the curtains. Indicate this.

Exercise 6.4: De-role

- *Outcome*
  Help participants to distance themselves from the role they were playing;
  Help participants to re-engage with the group as themselves, rather than from within the role they have just played.

- *Configuration*
  All participants in a role during the previous exercise.

- *Time*
  Five minutes.

- *Materials*
  None.

- *Process*
  All participants in the previous exercise stand in a circle with their arms around each other's waists.
  Each person in turn states: that they are not the person in the role they just played; their real name; where they are at that time; and something that is true about them at that

moment (e.g. what they are wearing, how they are feeling or what they are doing).

NB: It is important that everyone who took part in the role play should de-role before the plenary discussion of Exercise 6.3.

Plenary Discussion of Exercise 6.3a/b

- *Outcomes*
  Recognize elements of nonverbal communication within an 'everyday' scene;
  Identify the importance of nonverbal signals when communicating;
  Experience seeing oneself on video;
  Share thoughts and feelings about connections between participants' behaviour and the nonverbal messages;
  Share thoughts and feelings about watching oneself on video.
- *Configuration*
  The whole group.
- *Time*
  Approximately 40 minutes.
- *Process*
  The whole group watches the video of the role play once through, with the sound on and without comments from participants (this is to help to relieve the anxiety of seeing themselves on video).
  The facilitator then explains that the video will be watched through again, with the sound turned off.
  Invite participants to ask for the video to be stopped at any point where they may wish to make a comment about the nonverbal communication that has just taken place.
  The facilitators may also comment as appropriate.
  Tell the participants if it seems likely that you will not have time to go through the whole video.
  If time allows (after the tape has been rerun) encourage a free flowing discussion in which components of nonverbal communication not already addressed are discussed. Refer back to the 'brainstorm' material whenever possible.
  If no video is used, discussion focuses on the nonverbal signals used in each scene to portray a specific message (Table 6.1).
  If appropriate, facilitators might wish to restate the findings of Birdwhistell (1970) that 65% of all communication is nonverbal, and those of Hardin and Halaris (1983) that the types of nonverbal messages given most by 'high' empathy nurses are moderate

degrees of head nodding, steady gaze, smile, erect torso, a moderate number of gestures, and legs crossed but still, and those given most by 'low' empathy nurses are a high degree of head nodding, eye movements, laughing, frequent gesturing, torso movement, and leg movement.

NB: Allow about 40 minutes for the plenary discussion. For the role play without the video, discuss the same material as identified above.

Exercise 6.5: Warm Up – Hug-tag

- *Outcomes*
  Promote trust among participants;
  Sensitize participants to the use of touch as a supportive nonverbal signal;
  Energize the group;
  Have fun.
- *Configuration*
  The whole group.
- *Time*
  Five minutes.
- *Materials*
  None.
- *Process*
  The group pairs off, but leaves one member without a partner (if the group contains an even number of participants, the facilitator joins in the exercise).
  Each person then hugs his or her partner.
  When the person not paired up with someone else claps his or her hands, everyone must change partners, hugging a new partner. The person not paired up then attempts to find a partner, leaving another person alone.
  The new person without a partner claps his or her hands and the members of the group change partners again.
  This process continues until the facilitator calls time.

Exercise 6.6: Emotions and Nonverbal Communication

- *Outcomes*
  Help participants to identify nonverbal signals that may be associated with emotions;

Facilitate participants' recognition of differences between individuals in the interpretation of nonverbal behaviour related to emotional expression;

Encourage participants to examine the cultural element associated with nonverbal signals of emotional expression.

- *Configuration*
  Pairs (one group of three if there is an odd number of participants).
- *Time*
  Fifteen to 20 minutes.
- *Materials*
  Emotion cards;
  Flip-chart paper;
  Pens;
  Blu-tac.
- *Process*
  Participants divide into pairs and decide who is 'A' and who is 'B'.

  Person 'A' is given an emotion to enact nonverbally (from the list in Table 6.2: write each emotion word on a separate index card).

  Each person enacts (nonverbally only) the emotion on their card for two minutes in front of his or her partner.

  During this time, person 'B' is asked to observe the actual nonverbal signals displayed by person 'A' and write these down on large pieces of paper. Participants are asked to be very specific about the behaviours identified as nonverbal communication (e.g. eyebrows raised or hands with palms upward and fingers curling towards the body).

  At the end of two minutes, person 'B' is asked to write, underneath the behaviours previously listed, the emotion(s) they perceived person 'A' to have been illustrating.

  The partners reverse roles and 'B' is given a different emotion to enact and the previous process is repeated.

  When both partners have enacted an emotion, they share and discuss their findings within the pair.

  Subsequently, the papers are put up on the wall for discussion.

Plenary Discussion of Exercise 6.6

- *Outcomes*
  Examine the relationship between emotions and nonverbal signals;
  Explore cultural differences in interpreting emotions and nonverbal communication;

Table 6.2 Emotion words for index cards to use in Exercise 6.7

Sincerity	Warmth	Suspicion
Amazement	Approval	Attentiveness
Sadness	Sternness	Terror
Upset	Seriousness	Disgust
Distress	Anger	Pleasure
Rejection	Happiness	Disapproval
Pain	Disbelief	Threatened
Apprehension		Aggression

Examine possible misinterpretations of emotions because of observed nonverbal signals;
Share thoughts and feelings about emotions and nonverbal communication;
Share thoughts and feelings about misinterpreting emotions from nonverbal messages.

- *Configuration*
  The whole group.
- *Time*
  Approximately 30 minutes.
- *Process*
  The whole group re-forms to discuss the nonverbal elements of emotions that were identified during the exercise.
  Encourage individuals to focus upon the similarities and differences between nonverbal signals and emotions.
  Encourage discussion of individual and cultural similarities and differences in the way emotions are expressed nonverbally and subsequently interpreted.
  Ask participants to infer from the exercise the possible consequences for their own clinical practice.

Exercise 6.7: Evaluation of the Workshop

- *Outcomes*
  Help the participants to identify what they liked the most and the least about the workshop as a whole;
  Enable the facilitator(s) to identify parts of the workshop that might subsequently be altered;
  Allow time for participants to reflect upon the skills acquired and their practice.

- *Configuration*
  The whole group.
- *Time*
  Approximately 15 minutes.
- *Process*
  Each participant, including the facilitator, is asked to identify the one thing they liked the least about the workshop, or 'pass'.
  After all participants have responded, the facilitator asks each person to identify the one thing they liked the most about this workshop, or 'pass'.
  Participants are asked not to give or respond to any request for justification of their statements. They may also decline to give feedback by stating 'No comment' or 'Pass'.
  If used, evaluation forms can be given at this stage.

Reading List

Argyle, M. (1988) *Bodily Communications*, 2nd ed. Routledge, London.

McKay, M., Davis, M. and Fanning, P. (1983) *Messages: The Communication Skills Book*. New Harbinger Publications, Oakland, CA, pp. 59–69.

Rozelle, R.M., Druckman, D. and Baxter, J.C. (1986) Nonverbal communication. In *A Handbook of Communication Skills*. (ed. O. Hargie) Routledge, London, pp. 59–94.

Siegman, A.W. and Feldstein, I., eds. (1987) *Nonverbal Behaviour and Communication*. Lawrence Erlbaum, Hillside, NJ.

Chapter 7

Further Elements of Verbal Communication

In the course of evolution, humans have developed a complex system of communication that distinguishes them from all other members of the animal world (Ellis and Beattie, 1986). This system has evolved in an astonishing variety of forms and it is difficult not to be impressed by its sheer intricacy and beauty. However, not satisfied with stasis, human communication has capitalized upon its capacity for change. This makes it an infinitely flexible tool with which humans can communicate and reflect upon the ever changing nature of the world they inhabit. This workshop focuses on the elaborate and sophisticated elements of verbal communication.

Clearly, humans employ both verbal and nonverbal components of communication in order to interact with each other. These constituents of communication, in practice, are inseparable and the presence of both can enhance the clarity of messages. However, in a world where information plays an ever increasing role, verbal communication provides a dependable and flexible method of transmitting knowledge, concepts, feelings, theories and information (consider how difficult it would be to tell someone about your childhood using only nonverbal communication). Because this form of communication is essential when working with people in health care settings, it is vital that health care workers are able to use a variety of verbal communication techniques appropriate to the diversity of the situations in which they find themselves.

This chapter builds upon the verbal communication section of the introductory workshop in Chapter 5. It examines in greater detail the verbal element of communication and, as with previous workshops, contains a variety of structured exercises that will enable participants actively to engage in and explore issues related to verbal communication, including the effective transmission of information. It goes on to examine methods of questioning and responding to clients, and finally explores how communication may be categorized to increase its effectiveness in given situations.

Learning Outcomes

1. Recognize and use effective verbal communication techniques when responding to clients;
2. Recognize and use effective verbal communication techniques when questioning clients;
3. Practise using effective responding and questioning techniques in relation to the giving and receiving of information;
4. Utilize the theoretical framework of Six Category Intervention Analysis (Heron, 1989) when identifying verbal communication;
5. Share thoughts and feelings about the effective use of verbal communication skills.

Introduction to the Workshop

The facilitators need to state:

- *Learning outcomes for the workshop*
- *Methods used* Spend some time discussing this. Suggest that participation in the exercises will enhance learning and their enjoyment of the workshop, but let participants know that they will not be forced to take part if they do not wish to do so.
- *Time considerations* Make explicit the overall time for the workshop, and the time taken for breaks and when these might occur. Negotiate some flexibility in timing (up to 15 minutes either side of a stated time) but ensure that you finish on time.
- *Housekeeping issues* Locations of other rooms, toilet facilities, and eating and drinking arrangements; rules about smoking (e.g. designated areas, although we advise not to allow smoking during the workshop); issues concerning participants' safety, including fire procedures and those relating to personal items such as clothing, jewellery and footwear.

Exercise 7.1: Warm Up – Famous People

- *Outcomes*
  Enable participants to focus on the giving and receiving of verbal communications;
  Familiarize participants with the use of experiential exercises;
  Have fun.

- *Configuration*
  The whole group.
- *Time*
  Five minutes.
- *Materials*
  Cards;
  Sellotape.
- *Process*
  Each person chooses a famous person who they would like to be.
  Participants write the names of these people on index cards and attach them to their clothing.
  Members of the group then walk around, introducing themselves and responding as the character on their card. They also enter into dialogues with others to find out about them. Each person should attempt to meet as many people as possible in the time allowed.
  At the end of the period, participants de-role (see Chapter 1 on information relating to de-roling after experiential exercises).

Exercise 7.2: Verbal Information Giving

- *Outcomes*
  Practise using questioning and responding techniques to give and receive accurate information;
  Identify the role verbal communication takes in information giving and receiving.
- *Configuration*
  Small groups of three or four.
- *Time*
  Thirty minutes.
- *Materials*
  Blank paper and pencils;
  Copies of drawings (from Figures 7.1–7.4).
- *Process*
  Participants divide into groups of three or four, and allocate to themselves the initial roles of one 'planner', one 'artist', and one or two 'observer(s)'. (NB: All participants should have an opportunity to play all roles.)
  The planner and the artist sit back to back, with the observer(s) in a position to observe both of them.

The planner is issued with a drawing (Figure 7.1), which is kept hidden from the artist.

The artist is instructed to make a copy of the planner's drawing by obtaining information verbally (i.e. by asking *any* question they want). They may not face each other or share the picture. The drawing is made *solely* from the verbal description of the planner. The observer acts as arbiter of this rule.

The observer also listens to the types of verbal communication used, making notes if necessary, trying to judge the more effective types of verbal interactions.

After five minutes, the artist and the planner stop and share their respective drawings. The observer feeds back his or her comments about the verbal communication, whether it was effective or ineffective and why.

The participants change roles and repeat the exercise using a different drawing (Figures 7.2–7.4). After each turn, allow time to discuss the observations.

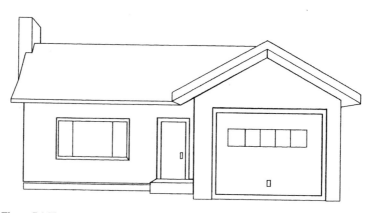

Figure 7.1 House

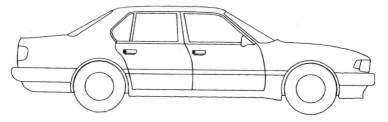

Figure 7.2 Car

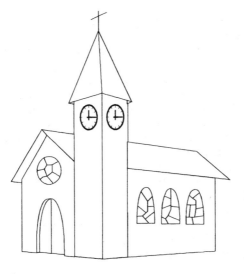

Figure 7.3 Church

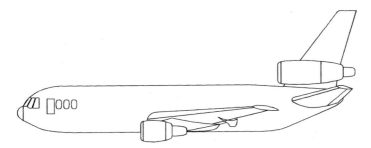

Figure 7.4 Jet plane

Plenary Discussion of Exercise 7.2

● *Outcomes*
  Identify the verbal communication that is used when giving information;
  Recognize the advantages and limitations of verbal communication when offering and receiving information;
  Identify barriers to effective verbal communication.
● *Configuration*
  The whole group.
● *Time*
  Approximately 30 minutes.

- *Process*
  The whole group reconvenes to discuss the effectiveness and limitations of using verbal communications only, when receiving and giving information.
  Facilitators encourage discussions about the need for accurate communication when giving information.
  Encourage a discussion about barriers to effective verbal communication and how they may be overcome.

Theory Input: Verbal Communication Techniques

- *Outcomes*
  Review verbal communication techniques in relation to questioning and responding;
  Explore participants' present understanding of verbal communication techniques;
  Identify examples of verbal communication techniques.

- *Configuration*
  The whole group.

- *Time*
  Approximately 15 minutes.

- *Materials*
  Optional use of overhead projector/white board to illustrate material.

- *Process*
  This section examines some verbal communication techniques (both responses and question), which, when used in the appropriate context, time, quantity and place, are skilled. However, some verbal communication techniques can never be considered skilled, while others are restricted in how they may be used skilfully. It is important for health care workers to be able to distinguish between the skilled and unskilled use of verbal communication, as skilled use is likely to be perceived as helpful to the client and further aid a good working relationship between the client and the health care worker.

Below are a group of skilled and unskilled questioning and responding techniques. Examples are provided for most of the skilled techniques.

Skilled Questioning Techniques

Open Questions

Open questions have no specific focus and invite clients to respond from their own frame of reference. They usually begin with words such as: What?, How?, Who?, Where?, When?, for example: 'What would you like to talk about?' or 'How does your condition affect you?'

Clarifying Questions

Clarifying questions aim to make clear the meaning of a client's statement. The questioner becomes increasingly focused upon the subject matter and begins to explore issues in depth, for example: 'What does having pain mean for you?'

Probing Questions

Probing questions enable the practitioner to explore more specific issues within the relationship. They are differentiated from open questions in that the subject tends to be of the practitioner's choosing, for example: 'How does the pain you are experiencing affect your mobility?'

Closed Questions

Closed questions are useful only for obtaining specific details, such as age, name, address, contacts, etc. They often elicit only a one- or two-word response (e.g. 'yes' or 'no'), and, as such, they should be used sparingly to avoid overwhelming the client. Often, such questions begin with 'doing' words such as: Have?, Did?, Is?, Can?, Are?, Would?, Could?, for example: 'Are you experiencing pain right now?'

Unskilled Questioning Techniques

Multiple Questions

This is asking more than one question in quick succession, which often results in the client responding to the last question only, for example: 'Were you in pain yesterday; or did you have a better day?'

Leading Questions

This is asking a question that assumes a specific response, for example: 'You are in a great deal of pain aren't you?'

NB: These questions may have some value when working with clients who have severe cognitive impairment that is unlikely to improve.

Closed Questions Inappropriately Used

This is using a closed question when an open one would be more appropriate or when the health care worker wants more than a one-word response, for example: 'Have you any pain in your head?' or 'Is it your head pain you would like to talk about?'

Skilled Responding Techniques

Echoing

Echoing is the repeating of the last word or phrase of a client's statement in a questioning tone of voice. It is used to encourage further exploration by the client of the issues raised, for example:

> *Client* This whole experience makes me feel unsettled.
> *Health care worker* Unsettled?

Reflecting Feelings

This offers to clients the practitioner's perceptions of the feelings that seem to be entwined within their verbal communication. Sometimes there may be a range of feelings and the practitioner will need to clarify what is uppermost for the client, for example: 'I sense that you are quite angry when talking about the pain you have.'

Paraphrasing

This is the rephrasing of the client's previous statement as the practitioner understands it, with a view to clarifying what is being said, encouraging further exploration of the issue, and demonstrating to the client that you are listening to him or her, for example:

> *Client* This pain sometimes makes me feel really tense, and I just feel like crying all the time.
> *Health care worker* It sounds as though what is happening to you makes you feel very unhappy.

Summarizing

This is the rephrasing of important aspects of the client's overall communication. Summarizing may include a client's statements from previous sessions. It can be used to clarify and review.

Facilitative Statements

These clarify what the client has said either verbally or nonverbally by the use of statements beginning with phrases such as 'I wonder . . .' or, 'I imagine that . . .'. They enable the client to perceive that he or she is being listened to and that the practitioner is aware of the feelings behind what the client is saying. Such statements do not imply or require a response, for example: 'I imagine all of this has had a considerable impact on your life.'

Validation

Validation is communicating to the client a genuine appreciation of his or her personal worth and value, without any qualification. It may be in relation to something the client has done or said but it may also simply be a means of valuing the client as a person, for example: 'You have made tremendous progress and I am impressed.'

Self-disclosure

Self disclosure is the *limited* sharing with the client of positive or negative thoughts, feelings and experiences from the practitioner's own life in order to demonstrate a level of empathy and understanding of the client's situation. Such a response must be used judiciously as it can be overpowering for the client and practitioner alike. It should be noted that even the physical presence of the practitioner is a source of self-disclosure, for example: 'I find I also get angry when things seem to be outside my control.'

Unskilled Responding Techniques

- Consistently ignoring the client's verbal (and nonverbal) communication;
- Being patronizing (i.e. speaking as if addressing a child rather than an adult;
- Being abrupt (i.e. offering only minimal verbal responses and speaking to the client with no warmth);

- Overinclusiveness (i.e. being verbose or answering in great depth a question that only requires a short response);
- Regularly interrupting the client's speech.

Exercise 7.3: Warm Up – Shaking Off the Dog

- *Outcomes*
  Begin to change participants' mental set from that of listening to being active;
  Physically restimulate participants;
  Have fun.
- *Configuration*
  The whole group.
- *Time*
  Five minutes.
- *Materials*
  None.
- *Process*
  Each person finds a space in the room.
  The facilitator asks each participant to imagine that they have a small dog tenaciously nipping his or her leg, and they must try to shake it off vigorously. The facilitator models this and encourages vigorous limb shaking by participants.
  After a few moments, the facilitator tells participants that the dog has now grasped the other leg and they shake that with equal vigour.
  Next, participants are told that the dog has attached itself to each of their arms in turn and they must try to shake it off.
  Finally the facilitator tells participants that the dog has jumped on their shoulders and must be shaken off.

Exercise 7.4: Verbal Techniques

- *Outcomes*
  Categorize verbal interactions;
  Identify the different effects that types of verbal interactions will have;
  Practise using specific questioning and responding techniques.
- *Configuration*
  Pairs (a group of three if there is an odd number of participants).
- *Time*
  Sixty minutes.

● *Materials*
  Flip-chart paper;
  Pens.

● *Process*
  Participants divide into pairs.
  Each participant will choose from the list in Table 7.1 a skilled
  communication technique that they would like to demonstrate.
  With their partners they prepare a role play demonstration of
  that skill, which will last for about 30 seconds for each participant.
  At the start of each presentation, the participant will state the
  technique being demonstrated, then demonstrate the technique
  with his or her partner.
  The partners in each group can enact a completely different scene,
  as long as the skill is demonstrated.
  At the end of each role play, other group members, including
  facilitator(s), comment on or ask for clarification of the technique
  just demonstrated.

Table 7.1 Verbal communication techniques

Skilled questioning techniques
Open questions
Clarifying questions
Probing questions
Closed questions

Skilled responding techniques
Echoing
Reflecting feelings
Paraphrasing
Summarizing
Facilitative statements
Validation
Self-disclosure

Plenary Discussion of Exercise 7.4

● *Outcomes*
  Recognize the need to use verbal communication that is context-
  specific;
  Share thoughts and feelings about the use of verbal communication techniques.

● *Configuration*
  The whole group.

- *Time*
  Approximately 30 minutes.

- *Process*
  Discuss the use of different types of questioning and responding techniques.
  The facilitator encourages reflection upon the rationale for using different forms of verbal communication therapeutically in different situations.
  The facilitator encourages discussion of the need for warmth and understanding when using verbal communication effectively.

Theory Input: Intervention Categories

- *Outcomes*
  Identify different categories of verbal skills;
  Offer a theoretical perspective to describe these categories.

- *Configuration*
  The whole group.

- *Time*
  Approximately 15 minutes.

- *Materials*
  Optional use of overhead projector/white board to illustrate material.

- *Process*
  When speaking with clients, whatever the health care setting, it is important that practitioners should interact sensitively. This entails being supportive and encouraging, while at the same time being noncollusive and, when appropriate, challenging. To do this effectively, the practitioner needs to demonstrate, through verbal and nonverbal communication, warmth and genuineness in the relationship, and an acceptance of the clients' beliefs, values, and feelings. One approach to the examination of these aspects of communication is through an analysis of the interventions that health care workers use with clients.

A model that can help health care workers to employ the most appropriate interventions with clients is the Six Category Intervention Analysis (Heron, 1989). These six categories are subsumed under two general headings: authoritative and facilitative. The former can be seen as more hierarchal and directive, while the latter tends to be more client led, with a focus on the affective aspects of the communication. It is important to recognize that neither type is 'better' than the other. However, some forms of traditional care environments tend to overuse authoritative interventions, while some of the newer ones may overuse facilitative interventions. An appropriate mix of both is generally thought to be the most beneficial.

Within these two groups are the six basic intervention categories, each with a number of specific interventions to enable helpful interactions between practitioners and clients. It is crucial to recognize that, when using particular interventions within these categories, this is done consciously and with a particular intention in mind, such as assisting the client to express unspoken emotions or clarifying the need for further information. Without this intention, the intervention is less likely to be effective and could also degenerate into an unhelpful intervention.

The two groups and six intervention categories are defined below.

Authoritative Interventions

Authoritative interventions involve the health care worker in taking some responsibility on behalf of the client to guide behaviour, give instructions, or raise consciousness. These are: prescriptive, informative and confronting interventions.

Prescriptive Interventions

Prescriptive interventions seeks to direct or influence the behaviour of the client so that some change may take place. They usually focus on behaviour outside the client–health care worker relationship. They may involve giving advice, persuading, making suggestions, or evaluating. They must be explicit, not vague, otherwise misunderstanding may occur. They could be interpreted as critical, especially if the intention is not for the client's benefit.

Informative Interventions

These interventions seek to confer knowledge, or give information or meaning to the client that has relevance to his or her needs or interests. Informative interventions are common in the helping professions, the members of which need to scrutinize how much information to give, or whether to give any information at all, and to facilitate clients in finding their own means of acquiring the information.

Confronting Interventions

Confronting interventions seek to increase the client's consciousness concerning some limiting attitude or behaviour of which they are relatively unaware. They directly challenge behaviour that is restricting the client within his or her personal and social world. Confronting interventions are not about conflict (i.e. they are not aggressive or combative). The essence is to heighten the client's awareness of the behaviour rather than coerce change. These interventions are also used when a behaviour is positive and the client's overall attitude is negative. The ultimate aim is to confront the pattern of behaviour *not* the person.

Facilitative Interventions

In facilitative interventions, the health care worker seeks to enable clients to become more autonomous and take more responsibility for themselves. This is accomplished by helping the client to release emotional pain, eliciting self-directed learning in the client, or affirming the worth of the client as a unique being. These are: cathartic, catalytic and supportive interventions.

Cathartic Interventions

Cathartic interventions enable the client to discharge or abreact painful emotions such as grief, fear or anger. The intention of these interventions must always remain conscious to the health care worker. The client must not be pressured to work at an emotional level beyond which he or she can contain. It is important that in all cases, when using these interventions, an explicit cathartic contract should be made. Health care workers also need to be aware that a client may have a cathartic experience as a result of a seemingly innocuous intervention, which may be the result of the client already being in a very emotionally charged state.

Catalytic Interventions

These interventions seek to help the client towards self-discovery, self-directed learning and problem solving. Their intention is to elicit a client learning process concerning how to live or handle feelings and reduce the effect of past trauma. With these interventions, the client develops insight into and understanding of his or her own personal and social processes, and what influences them. This results in self-directed discovery and self-generated change. These interventions are also used to encourage further exploration of clients' concerns.

Supportive Interventions

Supportive interventions affirm the worth and value of the client as a person, with individual qualities, attitudes, or actions, *without qualification*. Being supportive is an attitude of mind that underpins all health care worker–client relationships and is a precondition for all of the other interventions (i.e. one cannot inform or confront without being supportive). This, however, must be done without the health care worker colluding with the client's distortions, mis-identifications, inappropriate responses or defence.

Exercise 7.5: Identifying Interventions

- *Outcomes*
  Practise the identification of different types of verbal interactions using Heron's (1989) six categories;
  Practise the use of alternative interactions.
- *Configuration*
  Groups of three or four.
- *Time*
  Sixty minutes.
- *Materials*
  Flip-chart paper;
  Pens.
- *Process*
  Participants divide into groups of three or four.
  They have 10 minutes to construct a short scene in which one person is interacting with another.
  After the scene construction period, each group in turn enacts the scene to the other groups.
  During the scene, members of the other groups stop the action each time they can recognize an intervention within one of the Heron's six categories and state which category applies. (This may at first be experienced as disruptive, although, once participants become used to the format of this 'freeze frame technique', the flow usually picks up).
  After the scene, the participants de-role (see Chapter 1 for examples of de-roling techniques) and a short discussion of the intervention categories used is encouraged.

The next group then presents a scene and the process above continues.

After all the groups have presented their scenes and received feedback, a general discussion ensues.

Plenary Discussion of Exercise 7.5

- *Outcomes*
  Identify advantages and disadvantages of using Heron's (1989) six categories of interventions;
  Share thoughts and feelings about using the six categories of interventions.
- *Configuration*
  The whole group.
- *Time*
  Approximately 30 minutes.
- *Process*
  The whole group re-forms and the facilitator encourages a discussion of issues related to verbal interactions in general and the six categories in particular.
  The facilitator encourages a general discussion of the use of these interventions in health care settings.

Exercise 7.6: Evaluation of the Workshop

- *Outcomes*
  To help the participants to identify what they liked the most and the least about the workshop;
  To help the facilitator(s) to identify which parts of the workshop were liked by the participants and what parts might need revision;
  To offer the participants practice in giving negative and positive feedback.
- *Configuration*
  The whole group.
- *Time*
  Approximately 15 minutes.
- *Process*
  Each participant, including the facilitator, is asked to say one thing that they liked least about the workshop, or 'pass'.
  After all participants have responded, the facilitator asks each person to say one thing that they liked most about this workshop, or 'pass'.
  Participants are requested not to give or respond to any request

for justification of their statements. They may also decline to give feedback, but must state this (e.g. 'no comment' or, 'pass'). If used, evaluation forms can be given at this stage.

Reading List

Hargie, O., ed. (1986) *A Handbook of Communication Skills.* Routledge, London.

Heron, J. (1989) *Six Category Intervention Analysis*, 3rd ed. University of Surrey, Guildford.

Heron, J. (1990) *Helping the Client – a Creative Practical Guide*, Sage, London.

McKay, M., Davis, M. and Fanning, P. (1983), *Messages: The Communication Skills Book.* New Harbinger, Oakland, CA.

Chapter 8

Active Listening

Listening is an activity that is central to health care workers' repertoire of communication skills. For much of our time in clinical practice we are deluged with requests, entreaties, concerns, orders and advice. It is, therefore, little wonder that at times we defend against this by selective attention, or by listening but not reacting. However, when working with people, be they colleagues or clients, it is important for them to be able to recognize that they are being listened to with attention and understanding. Hence the need for what has been termed 'active listening'.

This chapter offers a workshop enabling participants to explore the concept of listening as a dynamic activity, and an opportunity to examine the differences and similarities between attentive and active listening, the former being a subset of the latter. It also offers an opportunity to acknowledge the feelings experienced when attentive and active listening do not take place. The workshop allows time for participants to practise skills, including listening actively to clients, concentrating upon the clients' verbal and non-verbal messages and identifying ways in which these messages might divert the health care worker's attention on to their own agendas.

The model of active listening presented is that of Watts (1986), which proposes three areas of the client's communication on which listening may be focused: 'manifest' content – the words used and their meanings for the client; 'reading between the lines' – the ability to identify alternative contexts within which the client's speech can be placed; and finally the 'latent' content – nonverbal messages and other material such as word choice, thematic repetitions, relative incoherence, or words and sentences that are said but not meant. However, what is also addressed in this workshop, which Watts (1986) does not discuss, is health care workers attending to or 'listening' to their own verbal and nonverbal communications.

Consistent with previous workshops, we offer a mixture of exercises, role plays, theoretical input and discussion. As with all workshops, we suggest a break after no more than two hours of teaching to allow participants to rest and reflect upon their experiences.

Learning Outcomes

1. Experience listening attentively to a client with only minimal vocal encouragers;
2. Share thoughts and feelings about the ease or difficulty of listening and being listened to without a verbal input;
3. Identify specific verbal and nonverbal components of active listening;
4. Experience the using of communication skills involved in active listening;
5. Share thoughts and feelings about the use of active listening;
6. Experience not being listened to actively;
7. Discuss, evaluate and give personal reactions to barriers to active listening.

Introduction to the Workshop

The facilitators need to state:

- *Learning outcomes for the workshop*
- *Methods used* Spend some time discussing these. Suggest that participation in the exercises will enhance learning and their enjoyment of the workshop, but let participants know that they will not be forced to take part if they do not wish to do so.
- *Time considerations* Make explicit the overall time for the workshop, and the time taken for breaks and when these might occur. Negotiate some flexibility in timing (up to 15 minutes either side of a stated time) but ensure that you finish on time.
- *Housekeeping issues* Locations of other rooms, toilet facilities, and eating and drinking arrangements; rules about smoking (e.g. designated areas, although we advise not to allow smoking during the workshop); issues concerning participants' safety, including fire procedures and those relating to personal items such as clothing, jewellery and footwear.

Exercise 8.1: Warm Up – London Bridge

- *Outcomes*
  Engage participants in the workshop;
  Enable participants to experience working together;
  Sensitize participants to the concept of listening;
  Have fun.
- *Configuration*
  The whole group.
- *Time*
  Ten minutes.
- *Materials*
  None.
- *Process*
  The group sits in a circle.
  The facilitator explains that he or she will say a sentence beginning 'I am going across London Bridge to . . .', and that each person in the group must repeat this in turn, adding their own destination. The facilitator will tell each person whether or not they can go to their chosen destination, the process being:
  The facilitator says, 'I am going across London Bridge to – er – Liverpool. I know I can.'
  Each person in the group is invited to repeat the phrase and add his or her own destination. Only if they include the 'er' before the destination can the facilitator say, 'You can.' Otherwise, the facilitator must say, 'You can't.'
  Go round the group several times until everyone has spotted the rule governing allowable destinations.
  Ask those who have discovered the rule to take over saying 'you can' or 'you can't'.
  At the end of the exercise, point out just how much information we all ignore when listening.

Exercise 8.2: Autobiography

- *Outcomes*
  Experience not listening to a section of someone's 'story';
  Experience not having a section of your 'story' listened to;
  Explore the thoughts and feelings associated with not listening and not being listened to, especially with regard to personal material;
  Reflect on the impact of not listening or being listened to in relation to interactions with clients.

- *Configuration*
  Pairs.
- *Time*
  Thirty minutes.
- *Materials*
  None.
- *Process*
  Participants divide into pairs and decide which person is 'A' and which is 'B'.
  'A' then begins to tell 'B' about aspects of his or her life in chronological order, going back as far as possible. 'B' takes an active part in the discussion, listening and clarifying as necessary. After three minutes, the facilitator asks all of the 'A's to change partners, finding a different 'B' to whom they continue to talk about their lives *from the point where they left off*.
  After a further three minutes, the facilitator asks the 'A's to go back to their *original partners* and complete their life stories, continuing from where they had just left off.
  Reverse the roles and repeat the exercise.
  The original pairs discuss:
    Thoughts and feelings about missing a section of someone's life story;
    Thoughts and feelings about not having the whole of their life story listened to;
    Identification of potential antecedents preventing a health care worker from hearing and listening to all of a client's story.

Exercise 8.3: Attentive Listening

- *Outcomes*
  Experience being listened to without interruption;
  Experience listening to another individual without interrupting;
  Practise nonverbal skills; this includes vocal encouragers such as 'mmm' that will indicate to the speaker that they are being listened to attentively;
  Practise listening unconditionally, without imposing any limitations or restrictions upon the speaker;
  Explore thoughts and feelings associated with being listened to and listening to a speaker attentively.
- *Configuration*
  Pairs.
- *Time*
  Fifty minutes.

- *Materials*
  None.
- *Process*
  Participants divide into pairs and decide which person will speak first.
  The speaker is asked to choose a topic that has an important meaning for him or her.
  The facilitator reminds participants of their obligation of confidentiality towards each other.
  The listeners' role is to listen attentively and, *without speaking*, to demonstrate their care, attention and understanding using nonverbal signals and cues (including paralanguage).
  After 10 minutes, reverse the roles and repeat the exercise.
  After a further 10 minutes, the pairs discuss what listener behaviours helped and hindered the speaker. The pairs also discuss their thoughts and feelings about the lack of verbal input from the listener.

Plenary Discussion of Exercises 8.2 and 8.3

- *Outcomes*
  Identify the feelings and thoughts associated with a part of your personal story not being listened to;
  Identify feelings and thoughts related to not listening to the whole of someone's personal story;
  Share feelings and thoughts about how this might relate to a participant's role in client care (e.g. sometimes what the client says triggers off personal thoughts of the health care worker).
- *Configuration*
  The whole group.
- *Time*
  Approximately 20 minutes.
- *Process*
  The whole group re-forms.
  Participants share and discuss particular issues that appeared important to them during the preceding two exercises.
  The facilitator asks participants to avoid discussing the actual content of the speakers' material, but to focus instead upon the benefits and drawbacks about not having listened to the *whole* of someone's story and of listening without giving verbal feedback, and also consider the impact that this might have upon client care.
  Participants share thoughts and feelings about being listened to and listening to each other.

Exercise 8.4: Defining Active Listening

● *Outcomes*
Gather material that might help to identify components of the concept of active listening;
Enable participants to define active listening from their general experience and that of the last two exercises.

● *Configuration*
The whole group.

● *Time*
Thirty-five minutes.

● *Materials*
White board and pen;
Large sheets of paper;
Marker pens.

● *Process*
The group elects one member to act as a scribe.
Participants spend five minutes gathering material, by stating ideas or words that have some meaning for them as individuals in relation to the concept of active listening.
During this period, the material is written down by the scribe on large sheets of paper.
Participants form into subgroups of four members and, using the material from the brainstorm, develop their own definition of active listening.
Each subgroup writes down their definition of active listening for presentation to the main group.

Plenary Discussion of Exercise 8.4

● *Outcomes*
Compare and discuss definitions of active listening from the subgroups;
Act as a precursor for the theory input from facilitator(s).

● *Configuration*
The whole group.

● *Time*
Approximately 20 minutes.

● *Process*
The whole group re-forms.
Each subgroup presents its definition of active listening.
The facilitator encourages a critical discussion of the advantages and drawbacks of each definition.

From the different subgroup definitions of active listening, the whole group produces a group definition, ensuring that the subgroup definitions are incorporated into the final one.

After the session, the facilitator offers some theory input on active listening.

Theory Input: Active Listening

- *Outcomes*
  Identify the value of active listening to improve client care;
  Identify one model of active listening;
  Recognize the process involved in listening actively.
- *Configuration*
  The whole group.
- *Time*
  Approximately 30 minutes.
- *Materials*
  None.
- *Process*
  Effective listening is an active process involving attending to communication (both verbal and nonverbal), processing and interpreting its meaning, recognizing and understanding its meaning for the client and conveying to the client (verbally and nonverbally) that you are in touch with what is being said.

  It is more than simply passive hearing. The listener's nonverbal communication, such as posture, movements, gestures, gaze and appearance, will have a key role in indicating to the client that the listener is listening to him or her. Conversely, the health care worker may prevent the client from feeling that he or she is being listened to and understood by exhibiting behaviours such as interrupting the client, allowing or responding to interruptions by others, appearing preoccupied with other work, and being overinformative or overprescriptive.

The model of active listening used here is based upon the work of Fraser Watts (1986). It suggests that active and effective listening consists of attending to three key areas of the client's communication. These are: listening to the manifest content of the client's speech; reading between the lines of the client's speech, and attending to the latent content of what the client is attempting to communicate.

Manifest Content

- This relates to listening to the words used by the client.
- It is an attempt to understand the meaning that the client may attach to words and phrases (and to *clarify* the meaning that the client may attach to those words).
- In doing this, it is necessary for health care workers to 'bracket out' their own assumptions about: the client as a person, the client's perception of his or her needs or problems, and the health care worker's own meanings of the words used by the client.

Reading Between the Lines

- Unlike attending to the manifest content, this involves the health care worker in making some assumptions about the meaning of the words the client uses, but always checking this out with the client.
- The health care worker needs to recognize the context of the client's communication (i.e. what the health care worker already knows about the client's history, the relationship that exists between the health care worker and the client, the client's understanding of his or her problems and needs, and the client's perceptions of his or her current situation and future).
- This involves identifying the issues being expressed by the client that have only minimal verbal or nonverbal evidence of what the client is actually trying to express. In these instances, health care workers concretize, through clarifying interventions, what seems to be implied by the client.
- The health care worker acts on the 'hunches' they have about the client's communication and checks the accuracy of these with the client.

Latent Content

- The latent content of the client's speech refers to verbal or nonverbal signals, which indicate issues and agendas that may be particularly significant to the client's well-being, but which the client may be unaware or unwilling to address.
- These signals are focused upon and fed back to the client at an appropriate point in the conversation to help to increase insight.
- Such indicators may 'leak out' in various ways. Watts (1986) suggests that the main ones include:

Moments of Unintelligibility

- *Affective* e.g. laughing after an emotional upset; shaking the head to mean 'no' when verbally saying 'yes'.
- *Cognitive* e.g. when the speaker's verbal expression begins to lose a coherent thread; made up words or phrases (neologisms) may be used; mumbling or a drop in the tone of the voice to the point where the listener cannot hear or understand a particular part of the conversation.

Sequence of Words, Phrases or Sentences

Abrupt changes in topic may be used as an unconscious or conscious avoidance of anxiety provoking material, for example:

Health care worker   You look unhappy today.
Client   When's lunch?

This can indicate anxiety about the health care worker's statement and a fear (either conscious or unconscious) of responding to it.

Slips of the Tongue

Psychoanalytical theory suggests that these are significant indications of possible inner conflict or an underlying important emotional meaning within the material that the speaker is conveying. It may also indicate contradictions between what people are saying and what they actually believe, for example: a British politician talking about the Anglo–Irish agreement and referring to it as 'the anguish agreement' (from a BBC radio news interview).

Use of Evaluative Terms

Often, indications of anxiety or conflict may be exhibited by the use (or overuse) of emotionally loaded descriptions of people or objects, for example: 'He must be absolutely and utterly the worst patient I have ever cared for in my entire career.'

Frequent or Repeated Use of Topics or Themes

Unconscious (and sometimes conscious) concern about a particular issue is manifested by the repetition of a particular topic or theme that the client wants to address, and perhaps does not know how to begin. The listening health care worker can pick up on such themes and introduce them into the agenda. For example, a client who uses various terms related to death and dying in the course of a single conversation may say, 'This ward is dead quiet... When I'm asleep I'm dead to the world... I'm just dying to get out of here.'

Active listening is also a combination of verbal and nonverbal elements of communication used by health care workers to encourage the client to communicate his or her thoughts and feelings because the listener indicates that he or she is attending to the whole meaning of the client's communication.

When actively listening to the client, it is important for health care workers to recognize the value of silence, either their own or that of the client. Using silence can reduce the possibility of negative behaviours such as interrupting and, with this, reduce the risk of missing important material that the client may wish to disclose. The client's use of silence also needs to be monitored in relation to the quality, length, timing and relationship to the verbal material that has been offered.

Exercise 8.5: Warm Up – Time Bomb

- *Outcomes*
  Help workshop participants to begin to concentrate on and process auditory signals;
  Re-engage participants in the workshop;
  Have fun.

- *Configuration*
  The whole group.

- *Time*
  Ten minutes.

- *Materials*
  Small box with a lid;
  Kitchen timer to fit in the box.

- *Process*
  Group members sit in a close circle (on chairs or on the floor).
  Set a kitchen timer or alarm to go off after 15–30 seconds.
  Place the timer in the closed box and instruct the participants to pass the box round the circle as quickly as possible.

When the alarm goes off, the person holding the box is deemed
to be out and must leave the circle.
Continue this process until the time is up or there is only one
person left in the game.

Exercise 8.6: Listening Triads – Building Active Listening Skills

- *Outcomes*
  Enable participants to experience using active listening effectively,
  encouraging the speaker to explore his or her own agenda;
  Enable participants to receive feedback on their use of active
  listening skills;
  Share thoughts and feelings on the ease and difficulty of active
  listening.

- *Configuration*
  Trios: speaker, listener and observer.

- *Time*
  Seventy-five minutes.

- *Materials*
  Copies of Table 8.1 and Figure 8.1.

- *Process*
  Participants divide into groups of three or four and allocate to
  themselves the initial roles of one speaker, one listener and one
  or two observers.
  Distribute copies of 'Topics for discussion' (Table 8.1) to assist
  the speakers in negotiating a topic for the exercise together with
  the listener (they can choose their own topic if that helps).
  The speaker and the listener conduct a 10-minute conversation
  based on the chosen topic.
  After 10 minutes, the listener summarizes (for 5 minutes) what
  has been said by the speaker.
  Both the speaker and the observer spend 10 minutes correcting
  any discrepancies in the summary and offering feedback on the
  effectiveness or otherwise of the listener's verbal and nonverbal
  behaviours in facilitating the speaker.
  Change roles and repeat the exercise until all participants have
  had an opportunity to be a listener.
  After each participant has had a chance to be the listener, the
  exercise is discussed in the small groups by:
  Distributing 'Questions for discussion' (Figure 8.1);
  Asking the participants to answer the questions and to write
  and discuss their answers prior to the plenary discussion.

Table 8.1 Topics for discussion

Capital punishment	Prison reform
Drug use/abuse	Ecology
Foreign policy	Political reform
HIV/AIDS	Rape
Feminism	Child abuse
Racism	Cohabitation
Euthanasia	Crime
Sexuality	Medical treatment

Consider the previous exercise for a moment, reflecting particularly on your performance in each of the three roles. Then write down your response to the question and statement posed below. You must wish to feed these back to the whole group during the next discussion.

What difficulties did you experience in each of the roles?

Speaker:

Listener:

Observer:

Identify at least three necessary components of effective listening:

1.
2.
3.

Identify something you learned about the effectiveness in your verbal and non-verbal communication while listening:

Identify three barriers to effective listening:

1.
2.
3.

Figure 8.1 Questions for discussion

Plenary Discussion of Exercise 8.6

● *Outcomes*
Examine the processes involved in effective active listening;
Identify helping behaviours in active listening.

● *Configuration*
The whole group.

● *Time*
Approximately 30 minutes.

● *Process*
The whole group reconvenes.
The facilitator encourages a discussion focusing on the responses made to Figure 8.1 in the small groups, scrutinizing:
What processes are involved in competent use of active listening;
What listener behaviours may hinder and encourage client interaction.

Exercise 8.7: Warm Up – Back to Back Talking

● *Outcomes*
Help workshop participants to experience being talked to while talking to another person;
Re-engage participants in the process of listening/being listened to;
Have fun.

● *Configuration*
Pairs.

● *Time*
Five minutes.

● *Materials*
None.

● *Process*
The group divides into pairs and each person sits on the floor, back to back with their respective partners.
Each person chooses a topic and begins to talk about that topic *at the same time* as their partner is talking about his or her topic. Participants are instructed to continue in this way for at least two minutes. They may also find it helpful if they are told that the key to completing this exercise is not to listen or to respond to each other.

Exercise 8.8: A Nonlistening Role Play

- *Outcomes*
  Help participants to experience having their own agenda to cover before examining what the other person is saying;
  Share thoughts and feelings about the emotions arising from not being fully listened to.

- *Configuration*
  Pairs.

- *Time*
  Twenty-five to 30 minutes.

- *Materials*
  Role play briefing sheets:

Client role: You live in a small rented flat in the city and have recently started working for a local firm. However, two days ago, the company went into liquidiation and you were made redundant.

You are now unemployed with very little money. Amongst your outgoings is your rent, which is due tomorrow. You are finding it hard to cope and the situation is making you very anxious and unhappy.

You finally decide to discuss your problems with a case worker at the local Job Centre, with the objective of getting help with your financial situation. You feel very upset and cannot waste time. You *must* make this case worker understand your predicament and its seriousness. You also believe that this case worker *must* be able to offer you practical help regardless of what they tell you.

Figure 8.2 Client role

Case worker role: You have been a case worker at a Job Centre for the past five months. One of the most difficult problems that you regularly encounter at work is dealing with clients who have very fixed ideas about what you can offer them.

Over time, you have decided that it is best to start discussions with clients by making it absolutely clear what you can and cannot offer. You can provide them with an opportunity to meet others in the same financial situation or a chance to discuss their problems generally. However you are *not* able to offer any form of practical help.

Thus, it has become part of your interview routine to make it clear to clients, before they make any assumptions, just what you are able to offer. If, in those initial stages of the interview the client attempts to ascribe more to your job than actually exists, you immediately put them right as to what you and the Job Centre can do.

Figure 8.3 Case worker role

Large sheets of paper;
Marker pens;
Blu-tac.

- *Process*
  The group divides into pairs and each person is given copies of the role play briefing sheets (Figure 8.2 and 8.3) and asked to spend a few minutes preparing themselves to enter the role described.
  Participants are asked *not* to share the roles with their partners until after the role play has finished.
  All pairs begin at the same time and each person enacts the role as described.
  The facilitator encourages participants to stay within role and to attempt to comply with all the instructions given to them.
  The facilitator stops the exercise after 10 minutes, or when the noise and frustration levels appear intolerable to participants.
  Each pair then lists their feelings and responses to each other at not having been listened to. These are written on a large sheet of paper for use in the plenary discussion.

Exercise 8.9: De-role

- *Outcomes*
  Help workshop participants to distance themselves from the role they were playing;
  Enable participants to relocate back into the workshop.

- *Configuration*
  The whole group.

- *Time*
  Five minutes.

- *Process*
  All group members stand in a circle with their arms around each other's waists or holding each other's hands.
  Each member of the group states that they are not the person in the role they have just played, states their real name, where they are right now, and something they are really going to do after the session.

NB: It is important that everyone who took part in the role play should de-role before the plenary discussion of Exercise 8.8.

Plenary Discussion of Exercise 8.8

- *Outcomes*
  Share thoughts and feelings in relation to their experience of
  conversations when 'turn-taking' is not involved and when it is
  involved;
  Share thoughts and feelings about practising the conscious use
  of questioning and responding;
  Share thoughts and feelings about the effect that nonverbal cues
  have on passing verbal messages accurately.
- *Configuration*
  The whole group.
- *Time*
  Approximately 30 minutes.
- *Process*
  The whole group reconvenes to discuss thoughts and feelings
  about not listening to each other's needs.
  Encourage discussion of issues such as:
  > Frustrations at not being listened to;
  > 'Competing' with another person to ensure his or her own
  > agenda was addressed;
  > Links between the levels of frustration they have felt and the
  > possible levels of frustration patients might feel in parallel
  > situations in health care settings.

  Facilitators should allow discussion of any other general issues
  relating to active listening and not being listened to.
  The list of further reading for this chapter can be given out at
  this stage.

Exercise 8.10: Evaluation of the Workshop

- *Outcomes*
  Help workshop participants to identify what they liked most and
  least about the workshop as a whole;
  Enable facilitators to identify parts of the workshop that might
  need alteration in the future;
  Allow time for reflection upon practice and skills acquisition.
- *Configuration*
  The whole group.
- *Time*
  Fifteen minutes.
- *Process*
  The whole group sits in a circle.

Each member of the group in turn states one thing they liked least about any aspect of the workshop. This can include facilitation, the material, the exercises or their own performance during the day.

Members may 'pass' at their turn but must not justify or respond to requests for justification of any statement they make.

After each member has responded or 'passed', then each member in turn states one thing they liked most about the workshop, or 'pass'.

Reading List

Argyle, M. (1983) *The Psychology of Interpersonal Behaviour*, 4th ed. Penguin, Harmondsworth.

Egan, G. (1990) *Exercises in Helping Skills: A Training Manual to Accompany The Skilled Helper*. Brooks/Cole, Pacific Grove, CA.

McKay, M., Davis, M. and Fanning, P. (1983) *Messages: The Communication Skills Book*. New Harbinger, Oakland, CA.

Nelson-Jones, R. (1990) *Human Relationship Skills*. Cassell, London, Chapter 5.

Smith V. (1986) Listening. In *A Handbook of Communication Skills*. (ed. O. Hargie) Routledge, London, Chapter 10.

Watts, F. (1986) Listening to the Client. *Changes*. (Jan), 164–67.

Chapter 9

Opening Interactions

By the time participants come to this workshop, we assume that they will already have developed a sound grasp of the basic components of communication skills and are using them effectively with clients. These health care workers may now wish to enhance their understanding and broaden the skills they have developed, including those associated with opening interactions. The way interactions are opened is important to all relationships and research has confirmed the old adage of first impressions influencing the development of relationships (Hampson, 1988; Leyens and Codol, 1988). It has also been suggested that the form that this initial contact takes can have a favourable effect on the development and growth of a healthy relationship (Berger, 1988) and that motivation to perform well can be dependent upon how communications are established (Sullivan, 1991). Health care workers, particularly those working in places where a large number of clients are seen in a relatively short space of time (e.g. clinic settings or accident departments), may be very reliant upon constructive strategies when initiating communications.

This workshop intends to offer an opportunity for participants to explore particular types of interactions that may be used to open communications with a client or group. The model presented is from the work of Christine Saunders (1986), who has clearly identified a number of ways interactions may be opened. Within this model it is recognized that opening an interaction does not only mean the first time a health care worker makes contact with a particular client. It can also mean the beginning of each contact in a series of sessions with a client or group, or a change in topic within the interaction. Ultimately, it is expected that health care workers should recognize and take into account a number of factors when initiating interactions or receiving them from clients.

Learning Outcomes

1. Experience opening interactions through introductions;
2. Share thoughts and feelings about the experience of opening interactions through introductions;
3. Identify the model used by Saunders (1986) for opening interactions;
4. Experience the use of different types of openings while role playing a health care worker–client interaction;
5. Share thoughts and feelings about the use of different types of opening strategies used in health care worker–client interactions.

Introduction to the Workshop

The facilitators need to state:

- *Learning outcomes for the workshop*
- *Methods used* Identify the teaching/learning methods to be used, suggesting that full participation will greatly enhance the learning outcomes, especially with the use of video recording equipment. Also obtain agreement from participants that personal material divulged during the workshop will not be disclosed outside of the group.
- *Time considerations* Make explicit the overall time for the workshop, and the time taken for breaks and when these might occur. Negotiate some flexibility in timing (up to 15 minutes either side of a stated time) but ensure that you finish on time.
- *Housekeeping issues* Locations of other rooms, toilet facilities, and eating and drinking arrangements. Rules about smoking (e.g. designated areas, although we advise not to allow smoking during the workshop). Issues concerning participants' safety, including fire procedures and those relating to personal items such as clothing, jewellery and footwear.

Exercise 9.1: Warm Up – Farmer, Fox, Chicken

- *Outcomes*
  Engage participants actively in the workshop;
  Enable participants to experience working co-operatively with others;
  Have fun.

- *Configuration*
  The whole group.
- *Time*
  Ten minutes.
- *Materials*
  None.
- *Process*
  The participants divide into two teams of equal numbers.
  The facilitator tells the groups that they will play one of three characters: farmer, fox or chicken.
  The facilitator tells the groups that each character has a special sign by which they are recognized: farmer – acting as if he or she has just fired a shotgun; fox – index fingers pointing up the side of the participant's head in a pretence of 'pointed' ears and looking furtively around; chicken – hands in the armpits, pretending to move his or her 'wings'.
  The members of each team decide which character they will be. There should be approximately equal numbers of each character within each team.
  The teams do not tell each other who is taking which character. The teams then line up along the wall on either side of the room. When the facilitator give the signal (e.g. says 'go'), the teams walk to the centre of the room and display their special signal to the member of the team who is opposite to them.
  The 'winners' of the display are as follows: farmer takes fox; fox takes chicken; and chicken takes farmer.
  The losing participants join the opposite team and the confrontations continue until all the members are lost from one of the teams, or the 10 minutes is up.
  The winning team will be the one with the most members left.

NB: This game can be played a number of times up to the allocated 10 minutes (although beware of overuse leading to growing disinterest or boredom).

Exercise 9.2: The Name Exchange

- *Outcomes*
  Practise initiating informative communication while listening actively to the information being given;
  Enhance the ability to focus on the communication being offered and not make assumptions from prior knowledge of the other person;

Reflect upon how initial contact is being made and its effect on the relationship;
Examine some barriers to listening to and responding to introductory interactions.

- *Configuration*
  The whole group.
- *Time*
  Twenty minutes.
- *Materials*
  Blank name badges;
  Blu-tac;
  Small (3 × 5 in) index cards;
  Pens.
- *Process*
  The facilitator identifies the outcomes for the session.
  The facilitator gives each participant a blank name badge, an index card, some Blu-tac and a pen.
  Each participant puts his or her name on the index card. This is fixed, with Blu-tac, on to the name badge, after which the participants wear it in a prominent place and walk around the room.
  The facilitator asks participants to introduce and exchange key pieces of information about themselves with another group member for approximately five minutes.
  The facilitator calls 'time' after five minutes and directs participants to exchange name index cards with each other.
  The facilitator asks participants to walk around and meet a person with another *name badge* and introduce and discuss themselves, for approximately two minutes, but *only* as the person whose name he or she is wearing (instruct participants to ignore any knowledge of the *actual* person whose name they are wearing).
  When the facilitator calls 'time', the participants switch index cards again and find a person with a different *name badge* to talk with, again talking only about the person whose name is being worn.
  This process continues until the facilitator calls 'time' after the total 20 minutes has elapsed.
  Finally, the facilitator asks each participant to retrieve his or her own name badge.
  Participants debrief the activity by making a short statement to the whole group about who they are, where they are, and the activity in which they have just participated.

Plenary Discussion of Exercise 9.2

● *Outcomes*
Discuss the experience of initiating an interaction that contains personal information;
Examine the types of opening strategies used;
Identify what may hinder accurate transmission and retention of information;
Discuss the need for effective introductory strategies in health care.

● *Configuration*
The whole group.

● *Time*
Twenty minutes.

● *Process*
The whole group reconvenes to discuss issues raised by the previous exercise.
The facilitator encourages a discussion of what may help or hinder the effective exchange of information.
The facilitator encourages participants to focus on the openings that occurred in the exercise.

Theory Input: Opening Interactions

● *Outcomes*
Explore the rationale behind opening interactions in particular ways;
Examine a theoretical framework for the opening interactions offered by Saunders (1986);
Discuss the effective/ineffective use of different interventions when opening interactions;
Recognize the context-dependent nature of using opening strategies competently.

● *Configuration*
The whole group.

● *Time*
Approximately 30 minutes.

● *Materials*
Handout of the five opening strategies, with sybtypes (Saunders, 1986):

1. Social: social reinforcement, establishing rapport, setting a receptive atmosphere;

2. <u>Perceptual</u>: environmental format, personal characteristics;
3. <u>Motivational</u>: initial behaviour, introduction of novel stimuli, posing an intriguing problem, making a controversial or provocative statement;
4. <u>Factual</u>: establishing a common frame of reference, stating one's role, goal-setting, summarizing;
5. <u>Client initiated</u>

- *Process*
  Before the theory input begins, distribute the handout to the group.

Introduction

The pattern of initial contact between individuals can foster or discourage the development of an open, facilitative relationship. Such encounters, when perceived as being warm and genuine, will enhance the progress of these alliances. Thus, to open an interaction in a way that is sensitive to the other person and the context in which it occurs, can increase the likelihood that such a relationship will continue and thrive. This is the type of relationship that is necessary for all health care workers, be they social workers, physiotherapists, social services staff, nurses, doctors, nursing home staff, volunteers, psychologists, etc., to function well enough in their role to address the needs of clients and others involved in their care.

Initiating interactions can serve a number of purposes, from beginning a relationship to changing the theme of a discussion. Goffman (1971) suggested that most interactions are purposeful, and may or may not be of benefit to those involved. However, the way interactions are opened can, unfortunately, be manipulative, either at a conscious or unconscious level. When consciously used, they have a malicious intent, as in the perverted interventions identified by Heron (1989). It is assumed that, within the setting of health care, interventions used to open interactions are designed to promote the well-being of clients and their carers. Operating on this premise, the reasons for examining how interactions are opened is to enable the beginning of a genuinely trusting relationship. The positive use of such interventions can strengthen this relationship and lay foundations for its future development. They can also be used in relation to acknowledging a perception the health care worker may have of the client and that person's environment (e.g. commenting on the smell of gas in the client's house, which can demonstrate a genuine concern). Other purposes may be to impart information, such as how much time is available for an interaction or to 'set the scene' (e.g. room layout) in preparation for the interaction, or when there is a change in the topic being discussed. Whatever the purpose, it is an important part of the interaction and prepares the individuals for the discussion. Recognizing the multiplicity of purpose for opening interactions, Saunders (1986) has suggested that they represent:

> ... the interactor's initial strategy at both personal and environmental levels, utilized to achieve good social relationships, and at the same time establish a frame of reference deliberately designed to facilitate the development of a communicative link between expectations of the participants and the realities of the situation (p. 176).

She also proposes that: 'There are a number of purposes for employing the skill of opening depending upon the duration and nature of the interaction' (p. 176).

It is these purposes, identified by Saunders, that will now be examined. The five opening strategies, with subtypes, have been outlined briefly in the theory input handout. The following is a more detailed account of these strategies. It is important to note that these are not presented as definitive or exclusive, but offer one set of strategies when considering how to open interactions more effectively.

Social Openings

This type of opening is used to begin the establishment of a facilitative relationship between the interactors. They help to establish and maintain a level of rapport that can enable the interaction to become a positive experience for all involved parties. They can allow a formal meeting to have the feel of informality without avoiding important issues that need to be addressed. These types of openings can also enable the participants to feel safe enough with each other to continue the interaction. Thus, social openings are important in maintaining a genuine, 'human' element in the interaction and to help to relax the client enough to begin to talk about difficult issues.

Social Reinforcement

This form of opening strategy is used to alert individuals to the wish to engage them in interaction, to begin that engagement, and to attempt to begin to hold their attention. This is done through a mixture of verbal and nonverbal signals. For example, attention may be gained nonverbally by the use of eye signals, such as directed gaze or an eyebrow flash. Other signals could be a smile while looking directly at the other party, a touch on a nonintimate part of the body such as the hand, or maintaining an acceptable distance. Verbal messages may be using a person's name or a verbal greeting, such as, 'Hello'. Both verbal and nonverbal messages need to be used in the appropriate context of the relationship between the individuals, such as social status, familiarity and the purpose of the contact.

Establishing Rapport

This type of opening is used most productively when the opening interaction signals the beginning of a relationship or it is recognized that there is a need to re-establish confidence in the relationship. They are often used in established relationships as a precursor to discussions about more substantive issues for the involved parties. Interactions that help to establish/re-establish rapport tend to be nontask orientated (e.g. comments on the weather or neutral comments about the news). This type of opening, however, can also be perceived as trivializing a client's problems if used when the client wants to get straight to the issues, if used too often, or if not delivered genuinely.

Setting a Receptive Atmosphere

This type of opening involves offering a psychologically and physically safe environment in which an interaction can develop effectively. On a practical level, it might be to ensure that the seating arrangements are satisfactory, there are no environmental distractions, or refreshments are offered if appropriate. On a less concrete level, it could be the health care worker setting the time boundaries, agreeing a contract of themes to be discussed, or establishing the level of confidentiality that will be kept during and after the encounter.

Perceptual Openings

When initiating contact with another individual, it is impossible not to perceive each other's surface characteristics and the environmental setting of the interaction. Therefore, in order to employ perceptual openings most effectively, health care workers need to be aware of their presentation and the environment within this initial contact. This can help them to choose the direction the interaction may need to take in order to facilitate the client's well-being. As well as health care workers being aware of themselves, they also need to be aware of the client and his or her environment. In consequence, this may involve presenting a potentially unpalatable perception to the client, the timing and strength of which depends on the relationship between the two and the reason for the challenge. Examples might be complimenting a client on his or her personal appearance when they do not feel they deserve such compliments or commenting upon disarray within a client's physical environment. Therefore, any perception, be it sound, odour, touch or sight, may become a focus, when appropriate, to use as a perceptual opening. Saunders (1986) has divided these into two main categories:

Environmental Format

At the time of face to face contact with a client, how the environment is perceived can affect the start of an interaction and its development. This could be the actual furniture used or its layout, ambient room temperature, colour schemes, light quality, etc. These can affect how the client or the health care worker perceives the encounter. If these environmental factors are within the control of health care workers, attention must be given to them in order to minimize disturbance to the client and increase the likelihood of a productive meeting. If control is not possible, however, then acknowledgement of this is important. Should the environment be one that the client controls, it may be appropriate to use an opening strategy that explores this environment and its relationship to the client. It is also necessary for health care workers to be aware of their own value systems and to what extent this may be affecting their perceptions of the client's environment.

Personal Characteristics

Influence on how an interaction may begin and develop is often a result of the characteristics of the interactors. Initial assumptions may be made by the individuals in the encounter because of physical characteristics, sex, race, style, voice quality, etc. This can affect how the interaction begins or new themes are addressed. Although these assumptions may alter over the course of the interaction or relationship development, there is always a danger that a stereotyping will occur and hinder the helpful progression of an interaction. Examples of this can be found in the attitudes of health care workers towards elderly clients or those of clients to health care workers' uniforms, such as general hospital nurses. Fortunately, such stereotyping is not usually persistent, as long as health care workers are aware of its occurrence.

Motivational Openings

This type of opening recognizes the need to stimulate clients in such a way that they will experience a need to participate actively in the interaction. It also focuses on the need to offer recognition that can motivate individuals to engage. Thus, attending to how a problem is addressed or a person presents themselves can increase the motivation of people to continue from the initial contact. There is also, on occasion, a need to change the stimulus in order to help to maintain attention and motivation. This is most valuable when health care workers are engaged in some form of education with clients. Thus, the types of opening strategies described as motivational are those that are more likely to increase the participants' ability to sustain attention throughout the interaction.

Initial Behaviour

This form of opening strategy is similar to perceptual openings in that its effectiveness is dependent upon how an action is perceived by the client. As specified, it would take the form of a behaviour (nonverbal or verbal) to initiate a discussion or simply to gain the client's attention in order to utilize another opening, such as a factual opening, in the early stages of an interaction. An example might be to place a hand on the client's arm or to call the person's name if he or she seems preoccupied and is not attending to the health care worker's presence. These interventions differ from social or other openings in that they are specifically aimed at motivating the client to attend to the subsequent set of interactions.

Introduction of Novel Stimuli

The introduction of novel stimuli is a well known technique in education circles for motivating students to maintain their attention within a lesson. In health care, the use of such a strategy may be helpful if the client is preoccupied with personal problems such as cancer, HIV infection or hallucinatory experience, or if the information being offered is too difficult for the client to understand at that particular time. Examples of these interventions might be for the health care worker to get up from the chair and stretch or to introduce booklets/pictures to offer a graphic, not just a verbal, explanation. It is important to note, however, that, when using this type of opening strategy, it must be handled sensitively and with caution, otherwise the client could perceive it as trivializing his or her problem.

Posing an Intriguing Problem

This type of opening may be used at the start of an interaction if the last meeting was left with an unsolved problem and the health care worker wishes to introduce the new session with this problem still to solve. More likely, however, is that the health care worker will hear a problem being posed by a client who intimates that there is no solution. The health care worker might then open up a fresh avenue of thought by restating the problem in a different way. An example of this might be a house surgeon being confronted by a client's despair at the prospect of a leg being amputated and how it might affect his marital relationship. The house officer, after listening actively and empathically to the client, might pose the question of how the client might respond if it was his or her partner who was losing a limb. Thus, the posing of such problems is aimed at the motivation of clients to identify part or whole solutions.

Making a Controversial or Provocative Statement

Within the context of health care, this type of opening strategy can usefully be made only after a satisfactory level of psychological safety and an effective relationship has been developed. It should not be used in new relationships. Such interventions are akin to paradoxical statements, where health care workers challenge the client's belief and value systems, which may be distorted. These statements are aimed at helping a client to open new and more healthy ways of thinking and feeling. An example of this may be in a therapeutic group setting when a group facilitator may challenge a client's statement that they are now more in touch with their feelings. Another example might be a social worker proposing to a client that he or she is not coping with a disability, contrary to what has been said by the client. Care, however, must be taken when using this form of opening intervention, as it can be interpreted as being patronizing or aggressive, resulting in the client becoming resistant, unco-operative or even hostile.

Factual Openings

A factual opening is used by interactors to ensure that both parties are clear about the purposes of the interaction, who is participating, what it is hoped will be gained, and how this might be achieved. As opening strategies, they help to prepare people for the discussion that is to follow by offering preliminary information pertaining to the individuals involved. They help the participants to know that their purpose for meeting and the issues to be discussed are congruent. This type of opening can also help individuals to clarify the goals they wish to achieve.

Establishing a Common Frame of Reference

This method of opening interactions is usually used at the start of the therapeutic relationship, often immediately following a short social opening. It establishes an understanding and agreement of what can be expected both in and from the interaction. There is usually an expectation that such an opening will confirm what one party can offer and what the other would like to receive (e.g. in the counsellor–client relationship).

Stating One's Role

This form of opening strategy performs a similar function to the previous one, but does so in a different way. Here there is some reliance upon the use of stereotyping. Thus, by stating one's role, any assumptions made by the other individual can be highlighted, resulting in a clearer idea of what to expect. For example, if a client is seen by a surgeon, just by having some knowledge of the surgeon's role, he or she will know that this individual has come to discuss the client's operation. The main danger in the use of this opening without further information is that stereotyping that has no validity may occur, resulting in erroneous expectations.

Goal Setting

When opening an interaction by facilitating the setting of goals, it is necessary first to have established some rapport with the client. Therefore, this opening method is often used at the start of a session in which preliminary information has been obtained or one goal has been achieved and it is time to begin to achieve another. This opening may also be the signal of a change in direction within an interaction from the assessment of needs to setting a goal.

Summarizing

Opening an interaction with a summary of what has previously taken place is one method of ensuring that both parties have a clear understanding of what has already been discussed and identifying their agreed route for progressing. Thus, any misunderstandings can be rectified. Interactions being opened in this way can clarify goals that still need to be achieved. Depending upon the interaction model being used (e.g. client-centred, behavioural, psychoanalytical, etc.), this strategy may be used at the start of each session or only at particular times.

Client Initiated Openings

This form of opening an interaction, although involving little verbal input by the health care worker, can often be the most difficult to use well. Although it often initially involves some form of short social opening, a requirement for silence from the practitioner is far greater. Thus, it necessitates a great deal of attentive and active listening (see Chapters 2 and 8 for further discussion of these topics). With this type of opening, the health care worker must wait for the client to begin the discussion or change the topic. As a result, the health care worker must avoid talking during a silence because of his or her anxiety, and must allow time for the client to begin. Occasional minimal encouragers, such as 'and . . .' or 'go on', may be given to demonstrate that the health care worker is attending, but it is important to let the silence continue until the client begins. Because this type of opening is so dependent upon the client to initiate the discussion, health care workers must obviously and genuinely show that they are attending fully to the client. It is also necessary for health care workers to choose the right person and time when using this type of opening. Such an opening adheres to the principle of client-centred care and is appropriate for use by health care workers who follow this approach.

Exercise 9.3: Role Play – Health Care Worker/Client

● *Outcomes*
Encourage the identification of opening strategies with clients;
Experience using particular strategies when opening interactions;
Differentiate effective from ineffective opening strategies;
Encourage participants to utilize the learning technique of video recording constructively during communication skills training.

● *Configuration*
Pairs.

- *Time*
  Depends upon the number of pairs; each scene requires approximately 15 minutes, consisting of: five minutes for preparation; 10 minutes for the role play.
- *Materials*
  A room large enough to accommodate the participants in a role play plus observers;
  Video camera, video recorder and television monitor (set up for display prior to the start of the workshop);
  Observer prompt sheet (see Table 9.1).

Table 9.1 List of opening strategies

Social openings	Social reinforcement
	Establishing rapport
	Setting a receptive atmosphere
Perceptual openings	Environmental format
	Personal characteristics
Factual openings	Establishing a common frame of reference
	Stating one's role
	Goal setting
	Summarizing
Client initiated openings	

Role play profile sheets:

Profile 1: Client
    You are 22 years old and have lived at home with your parents since leaving school. You had a variety of jobs but none has suited you and you are currently unemployed. You have no friends.
    Because of this you have begun to feel very low in mood and tearful at times. You do not feel that life is very worthwhile and have thoughts of killing yourself, although you have made no particular plans.
    You know that your mother is very worried about you and that she has talked to your GP. Your mother tells you that 'someone' is going to come to see you.
    You have been in your bedroom and now hear the front doorbell ring, shortly followed by a knock at your bedroom door. Answer it.

In this role play, try to be quiet and withdrawn without being hostile. Avoid communication without being rude. Try to assess the opening interventions. Do they help you to feel like talking?

Profile 1: Health care worker
You are a locum GP who has been asked to see a patient because his mother is frightened and very worried.

The only details you have is that the client is aged 22, has lived with his/her parents all his/her life and that since leaving school he/she has had a variety of jobs but is now unemployed. The mother is apparently very worried because your client has become very withdrawn and spends most of the day in his/her bedroom.

You arrive and are admitted by the mother. Her son/daughter is in the bedroom. You go upstairs at once and knock on the door.

In this role play, use appropriate opening interventions in an attempt to gain the client's confidence. Try to help him/her to feel able to talk with you.

Profile 2: Client
You have recently been discharged from a psychiatric hospital where you had been compulsorily detained because it was said that you had been behaving oddly and were considered dangerous to others.

Your stay was only for one month, but you feel quite resentful about having been kept there. You are glad to be home and now feel very well, although sometimes people irritate you by staring at you when you walk down the street.

You are in the sitting room of your house when there is a knock on the door. You answer it.

In this role play, you should appear to be hostile and argumentative without being violent. Try to assess to what extent the opening interactions help you to become calm and receptive or to remain hostile.

Profile 2: Health care worker
You are a community psychiatric nurse attached to a hospital-based service. You have been asked by the ward team to see a client who was discharged from hospital three weeks ago following a month-long admission under the Mental Health Act 1983 for treatment of a paranoid illness.

While your client was an inpatient, the doctors prescribed depot medication, which was started on the ward. You met the client on the ward and it seemed that, although reluctant, he/she was willing to see you at home to continue medication.

You arrive at the patient's house and knock on the door.

In this role play, try to use opening interactions to strengthen the relationship you formed some weeks back. Be aware of which openings seemed to help and those that seemed to hinder the interactions.

Profile 3: Client

You are about to be discharged from hospital after a recurrent episode of pneumonia. The nursing and medical staff have expressed their concern about your home situation. They have suggested that it will be hard for you and your wife to cope in your first floor flat considering your chronic breathing difficulties. You, however, take a different view and have stated categorically that you have lived there for the past 65 years and will be fine for another 65 years.

The charge nurse has now informed you that a social worker will be visiting you to discuss the possibility of some form of alternative accommodation. Although you are very polite, inside you are thinking things such as: 'They'll put me in an old people's home', 'What will happen to my wife?', 'They are going to take everything away from me and my wife', plus more. In the back of your mind, you realize you both need some help but you are frightened and angry at the possibility that your independent life will be destroyed.

While you are sitting in the communal area, someone approaches you and introduces him/herself.

In this role play, try to maintain a semblance of politeness while still feeling a mixture of fear and anger. Be co-operative but adamant about your position of wanting to remain totally independent. Try to assess how the opening interactions of the social worker have helped you to control your feelings, and also what, in the opening moments of the interaction, helped or hindered you in holding a conversation with him/her.

Profile 3: Health care worker

You are a busy social worker with a large case load. One of your clients, who you have known for four years and who is on your files, has suffered from chronic bronchitis for the past 10 years. At least twice each winter he requires admission to hospital. You know that each time he leaves hospital he deteriorates more and has increasing difficulty with his mobility. You also recognize that his wife seems to be having problems in coping alone with his needs.

You have been contacted by the ward charge nurse who discusses the nursing and medical staff's concern about his living conditions. You are told that this was precipitated by his imminent discharge and the present shortage of beds for more acute clients.

You go to the ward to discuss this matter with him and find him in the common room.

During this role play, use opening interactions skills to attempt to set the scene so that you can assess the person's needs and how they may be feeling. Try to assess which openings help you most and which hinder the conversation.

Profile 4: Client
You are a permanent resident in a nursing home for people with a variety of physical disabilities. Your disability is spina bifida; you are catheterized and confined to a wheelchair. You enjoy outdoor activities and reading. Occasionally you become verbally abusive, although seem to be unaware of this at the time. You have recognized that you get frustrated at your limited movement and frequent reliance on others to help you get around. You have often said to people in the house that your mother does not show much concern for you. Your father died one year ago and you were unable to attend his funeral.

A new worker started at the home last week. You want to get to know him/her but are afraid to do so. He/she has observed you in a verbally aggressive outburst and you do not know his/her reaction, but would like to know. Sometimes you are withdrawn but usually you engage in normal conversation.

This new worker now approaches you in an attempt to get to know you.

In this role play, try to portray the feelings of fear and frustration you have. Do not seek to initiate conversation but be prepared to respond if you feel the worker does show some interest in you as a person. In addition, try to assess to what extent the opening interactions used by the worker helped you to communicate your feelings.

Profile 4: Health care worker
You are a new member of staff at a nursing home that cares for clients with a variety of physical disabilities. Your experience in health care is limited although you want to learn as much as possible because it is an area that interests you. You have met

most of the clients by now but there are still two left to meet. You are determined to have talked with everyone at least once by the end of your first week.

There is one person, who has spina bifida and is confined to a wheelchair, whom you have not talked with yet. This client generally seems pleasant, although you have witnessed one verbally abusive outburst. This has made you a bit uncertain about how to approach him/her, but your determination and wish to develop some form of relationship with all residents spurs you on. You feel certain that once you get to know this person you will understand the outburst.

You now approach this person in the day room to have your first conversation.

During this role play, try to use skills to open the interactions that seem appropriate in getting to know the client. Try to assess which of these skills help or hinder you in starting and continuing the conversation.

● *Process*

Participants are asked to form into pairs (one participant may need to play a client twice if there is an odd number of participants).

Each participant is given a role play profile of either a client or a health care worker.

Participants are then given approximately five minutes to look at their role play profile, ensuring that they do not show their profile sheets to their partners.

All role play scenes are videoed in turn, with a discussion being undertaken after *all* of the scenes are finished (unless video equipment is not available or participants adamantly refuse to use the video).

All nonparticipants of each role play scene will be given an observer prompt sheet to complete for the discussion later.

The observer's task is to identify as many of the components of the openings as they can – writing down where they took place in the scene – to be presented during discussion of the videos.

After all scenes are enacted, the whole group de-roles.

NB: The health care worker in the role play profile sheets, as in all role play settings in this book, is considered to be an occupational therapist, a physiotherapist, a nurse, a social worker, a doctor, a psychologist, a care assistant, or any other employee/volunteer whose remit is to care for people with health needs.

Exercise 9.4: De-role

- *Outcomes*
  Help participants to distance themselves from the role they were playing;
  Help participants to re-engage with the group as themselves rather than from within the role they have just played.

- *Configuration*
  All participants in a role from the previous exercise.

- *Time*
  Five minutes.

- *Materials*
  None.

- *Process*
  All participants in the previous exercise stand in a circle with their arms around each other's waists.
  Each person, in turn, states that they are not the person in the role they have just played, states their real name, states where they are right now, and states something that is true about them at that moment (e.g. what they are wearing, how they are feeling or what they are doing).

NB: It is important that everyone who took part in the role play should de-role before the plenary discussion of Exercise 9.3.

Plenary Discussion of Exercise 9.3

- *Outcomes*
  Explore strategies used when opening interactions with clients;
  Identify the types of openings used and when they were used, based on information from the observer prompt sheets;
  Discuss thoughts and feelings about methods and outcomes when using different types of opening strategies.

- *Configuration*
  The whole group.

- *Time*
  Approximately 45 minutes, depending on the number of participants.

- *Process*
  The whole group reconvenes to watch each video sequence and discuss issues raised in them.

As each video scene is watched, pause when either a group member or a facilitator identifies a discussion point.

When an opening interaction is identified on an observer prompt sheet, that observer may ask to stop the video to highlight the strategy used.

Encourage participants to discuss what may help or hinder a constructive opening from taking place.

Facilitators should encourage discussions of helpful interactions only and ignore less useful ones, unless an absolutely dangerous practice is observed.

Focus the discussion on using video recording as a positive learning experience.

If video equipment was not used, the same process can be followed, or short discussions can be facilitated after each of the role play scenes.

Exercise 9.5: Evaluation of the Workshop

- *Outcomes*
  Help the participants to identify what they liked most and liked least about the workshop as a whole;
  Enable the facilitator to identify parts of the workshop that might be altered in future;
  Allow time for participants to reflect upon the skills acquired and their practice.
- *Configuration*
  The whole group.
- *Time*
  Approximately 15 minutes.
- *Process*
  Each participant, including the facilitator, is asked to say one thing they liked least about the workshop, or 'pass'.
  After all participants have responded, the facilitator asks each person to say one thing they liked most about this workshop, or 'pass'.
  Participants are requested not to give or respond to any request for justification of their statements. They may also decline to give feedback by stating 'No comment', or 'Pass'.
  If used, evaluation forms can be given at this stage.

Reading List

Culley, S. (1991) *Integrative Counselling Skills in Action*. Sage, London.

Heron, J. (1989) *Six Category Intervention Analysis*, 3rd ed. (Human Potential Research Project.) University of Surrey, Guildford.

Saunders, C. (1986) Opening and closing. In *Communications Skills*. (ed. O. Hargie) Routledge, London, Chapter 7.

Chapter 10

Sustaining and Controlling Interactions

Throughout these workshops, we have indicated that a significant feature of effective communication is to enable clients to help themselves whenever possible. This empowerment necessitates the development of a nondirective, facilitative approach to communication rather than a prescriptive, 'doing unto' method. However, there are also times when health care workers need to take a more prominent role within a relationship in order to sustain interactions or possibly control those that have become countertherapeutic. For example, occasions might arise when a client is very withdrawn and the health care worker needs to be more proactive in maintaining the communication between them until such a time as the client can initiate interactions. Conversely, while control within an interaction will naturally shift between the client and the health care worker, there are occasions when the health care worker will need to gain control. An example of this might be when a client is unable or unwilling to discontinue the flow of speech or behaviour because of very high levels of anxiety and may need some direction from the health care worker to re-establish control and thus communicate effectively.

This workshop focuses on the skills of sustaining and, when appropriate, controlling interactions with clients. It builds on the skills of active listening explored in Chapter 8, in particular, how listening to the latent content of a client's communication can enable the health care worker to identify the emotional content of a client's speech or behaviour, indicating potential avenues to follow in sustaining momentum in the interaction. For example, the actual words used by clients may indicate an emotional loading in what is being conveyed verbally. It is this, as well as the nonverbal material that the client is projecting, that can help health care workers to recognize which areas of communication to focus their energies upon to help to sustain therapeutic interactions. Additionally, this workshop offers time to explore the potentially difficult issue of controlling an interaction, and enables participants to develop and practice one technique that can be used in controlling an interaction therapeutically.

Learning Outcomes

1. Experience and identify the effect that the emotional content of verbal and nonverbal communication can have on sustaining interactions;
2. Share thoughts and feelings about how the emotional content of words and/or behaviour may affect sustaining and controlling interactions;
3. Experience and identify the part played by catalytic and cathartic interventions in sustaining and controlling an interaction;
4. Practise skills associated with catalytic and cathartic interventions;
5. Experience controlling an interaction therapeutically by using the technique of 'Talk-over';
6. Share thoughts and feelings about using such a technique.

Introduction to the Workshop

The facilitators need to state:

- *Learning outcomes for the workshop*
- *Methods used* Identify the teaching/learning methods to be used, suggesting that full participation will greatly enhance the learning outcomes. Also obtain agreement from participants that personal material divulged during the workshop will not be disclosed outside the group.
- *Time considerations* Make explicit the overall time for the workshop, and the time taken for breaks and when these might occur. Negotiate some flexibility in timing (up to 15 minutes either side of a stated time) but ensure that you finish on time.
- *Housekeeping issues* Locations of other rooms, toilet facilities, and eating and drinking arrangements; rules about smoking (e.g. designated areas, although we advise not to allow smoking during the workshop); issues concerning participants' safety, including fire procedures and those relating to personal items such as clothing, jewellery and footwear.

Exercise 10.1: Warm Up – Structures

● *Outcomes*
Encourage creativity;
Assist participants to engage in the workshop;
Enable participants to experience working together and being in close contact with each other;
Sensitize participants to each other's nonverbal signals;
Have fun.

● *Configuration*
Small groups.

● *Time*
Ten minutes.

● *Materials*
None.

● *Process*
Divide into small groups of no more than six participants. Each group must work as far away from the others as possible to avoid distraction.
Each group spends five minutes devising a structure, which they make using only their own bodies. Structures may be any *real* object (e.g. Leaning Tower of Pisa, Arc de Triomphe, Tower Bridge, a church, a car, etc.
After five minutes, the whole group reconvenes and each small group demonstrates their structure to the others.
Members of the other groups try to guess what the structure represents.

Exercise 10.2: Emotional Loading with Words and Nonverbal Signals

● *Outcomes*
Encourage participants to listen to the latent content of speech (see Chapter 8 for definition of latent content);
Experience and identify feelings evoked by particular words;
Identify how voice tone and speed, gesture, body movement and posture may positively or negatively affect the listener's perception of communication;
Reflect on the impact of nonverbal cues in relation to the emotional content of communication;
Share thoughts and feelings concerning the impact that nonverbal signals may have upon the emotional content of communication.

- *Configuration*
  Pairs.
- *Time*
  Thirty minutes.
- *Materials*
  Handouts (Tables 10.1–10.4);
  Pencil and paper.
- *Process (in two parts)*
  Part A (*Tables 10.1 and 10.2*)
  The group separates into pairs; each pair decides who takes the role of the listener and the role of the reader.
  The reader is given a list of affectively negative words (Table 10.1) and, following the instructions on the sheet, reads these aloud to the listener.
  The listener reflects upon the feelings that those words evoke and writes them down.
  When the reader has finished, the listener leads a discussion for five to 10 minutes, identifying the feelings associated with those words. Both participants attempt to identify what may have influenced the experiencing of these feelings.
  The roles are reversed and the new reader is given a list of affectively positive words (Table 10.2), which he or she reads aloud to the new listener, following the instructions on the list.
  The listener reflects upon the feelings that these words evoke, writing them down and leading a discussion for five to 10 minutes on the feelings associated with these words. Again, both participants attempt to identify what may have influenced the evocation of these feelings.

  NB: It is important to instruct participants *not* to reveal the list of words or their emotional loading until after the whole exercise is completed.

  Part B (Figures 10.3 and 10.4)
  Participants form into different pairs to those in the previous exercise; each pair decides who takes the role of the listener and the role of the reader.
  The reader is given a list (list 1) of affectively neutral words (Table 10.3) and reads these out loud to the listener, following the instructions on the sheet explicitly.
  The listener reflects upon the feelings that those words evoke and writes them down.
  When the reader has finished, the listener leads a discussion for five to 10 minutes, identifying the feelings associated with those

Table 10.1 Affectively negative words
The following words can all be classed as affectively negative. Your task is slowly to read out all of the words to your partner, in an as neutral and unemotional way as possible. Try not to convey any feelings in your voice or behaviour. At the end of the list, your partner will describe the feelings that the words convey.

NB: Do not show this list to your partner or indicate the affective loading of the words.

Forget	Curse
Cretin	Dissolve
Hard	Consume
Monster	Disappear
Horror	Hideous
Destroy	Pain
Erode	Wrong
Death	Pitiful
Devoid	Black
Weird	Lament

Table 10.2 Affectively positive words
The following words can all be classed as affectively positive. Your task is slowly to read out all of the words to your partner, in an as neutral and unemotional way as possible. Try not to convey any feelings in your voice or behaviour. At the end of the list, your partner will describe the feelings that the words convey.

NB: Do not show this list to your partner or indicate the affective loading of the words.

Breeze	Sweet
Friendly	Spirit
Glory	Green
Slender	Garden
Musical	Grace
Fawn	Life
Silver	Clear
Tranquil	Rest
Light	Majestic
Fluffy	Growing

words. Both participants attempt to identify what may have influenced the evocation of these feelings.

The roles are reversed and the new reader is given another list (list 2) of affectively neutral words (Table 10.4) which he or she

Table 10.3 Affectively neutral words (list 1)
The following words are all classed as affectively
neutral. Your task is to read these words slowly to
your partner, in such a way as to convey either *positive*
or *negative* feelings, using *only* appropriate gestures,
body movements, posture, and voice tone and speed.
    NB: Do not tell your partner verbally what feelings
you intend to convey.

You	If
Is	Has
For	That
All	The
A	Thus
On	Which
From	By
What	Now
With	Except
Unless	But

reads aloud to the new listener, following the instructions on the list.

The listener reflects upon the feelings that these words evoke, writing them down and leading a discussion for five to 10 minutes, after the reader has finished focusing upon the feelings associated with these words. Again, both participants attempt to identify what may have influenced the evocation of these feelings.

NB: Again it is important to instruct participants *not* to reveal the list of words or the expected emotional implications of the nonverbal signals until after the whole exercise is completed.

Plenary Discussion of Exercise 10.2

- *Outcomes*
  Share thoughts and feelings about how word choice can influence the emotional tone of an interaction;
  Share thoughts and feelings about how nonverbal signals can influence the emotional tone of an interaction.
- *Configuration*
  The whole group.
- *Time*
  Approximately 30 minutes.
- *Process*
  The whole group reconvenes to discuss issues raised by Exercise 10.2.

Table 10.4 Affectively neutral words (list 2)
The following words are all classed as affectively
neutral. Your task is to read these words slowly to
your partner, in such a way as to convey either *positive*
or *negative* feelings, using *only* appropriate gestures,
body movements, posture, and voice tone and speed.
NB: Do not tell your partner verbally what feelings
you intend to convey.

It	Though
Some	This
Those	Out
To	Where
Them	Words
About	Into
Or	Over
And	As
Are	Therefore
When	One

The facilitator encourages or, if necessary, introduces issues such as:

How the choice of words can influence the affective meaning of an interaction;

The effect of nonverbal communication upon the affective perception of words.

Theory Input: Catalytic and Cathartic Interventions

● *Outcomes*
Identify affective aspects of communication;
Examine the meaning of catalytic and cathartic interventions;
Identify some skills associated with catalytic and cathartic interventions.

● *Configuration*
The whole group.

● *Time*
Approximately 15 minutes.

● *Materials*
None.

● *Process*
Some level of emotional bias is often implied by particular words, intimating favourable or unfavourable attitudes (Philbrick, 1966). Whether this results from an internal mechanism or just external

stimuli (or both) can be argued. However, in support of the external stimuli hypothesis, it has been suggested that cultural and social influences on communications can alter their meanings and perceived emotional content (Izard, 1980; Slobin, 1979). Being aware of this and responding therapeutically to the emotionally laden content of a client's speech can help to sustain interactions and move them forward. Techniques using skills associated with catalytic and cathartic interventions (Heron, 1990) are a means of supporting and nourishing interactions that require encouragement to continue.

Cathartic Interventions

Cathartic interventions facilitate the release of tensions and the expression of distress associated with the unleashing of often painful emotions such as anger, grief, fear or embarrassment. The client may discharge emotions by sounds and movements, tears and sobbing, trembling and shaking, or laughter. Sometimes, however, the client is in such distress that any empathic intervention will bring about a cathartic release. Generally, the health care worker will rely on active listening skills in order to detect distressing emotional material that the client may be experiencing.

Because of the power of cathartic interventions, it is vital to obtain an explicit agreement from the client to work on this emotional material prior to commencement. There are times, however, when a cathartic release may occur with little or no prior indication of the effect an intervention may have on a client. When painful material does surface, the health care worker may choose to work with the 'content cues' of what the client is saying, or with the 'process cues' (Heron, 1990).

Content cues are *what* the client is saying: the meanings, stories and images that a client uses. Heron suggests that interventions that focus on content include:

- *Giving permission* Initially, clients may find it very difficult to discharge distress, perhaps because of social conditioning. In giving verbal permission and encouragement to the client, the health care worker enables the commencement of emotional discharge.

- *Present tense accounts* The client is asked to relate particular incidents as though they are happening in the present. This also includes intervening when the client starts to use the past tense, in order to bring the incident back into the present.

- *'What's on top?'* The client is invited to state what experience, however trivial or remote, comes spontaneously to mind.
- *Validation* This is genuinely affirming the worth of the client in order to contradict his or her negative self-image.

Process cues are those manifestations of *how* the client is talking and behaving. They may include the volume and tone of the voice, breathing, facial expression, gestures and posture. Interventions that focus on process include:

- *Repetition* The health care worker asks the client to repeat emotionally charged words or phrases, perhaps repeating them louder and louder. Small movements that may indicate distress can also be a focus and be managed in the same way.
- *Touch* Reaching out to touch lightly, hold or hug the client can help to facilitate the commencement or intensification of catharsis.
- *Pursuing the eyes* When a client avoids eye contact, perhaps to avoid facing distress, the health care worker precipitates or continues catharsis by gently pursuing the eyes of the client, if necessary looking up at them if the client's head is lowered.

When using cathartic interventions, it is important for the health care worker to pitch the level and depth of the intervention to his or her perception of the client's needs, in order to avoid overwhelming the client. Thus, using these interventions before the client is ready, or using those that encourage more emotional release than the client can withstand at that moment, may result in the client further suppressing painful material. Any spontaneous verbalization of insight from the client may happen quickly or over a long time period. Thus, health care workers need to ensure that there is time for the client to reflect upon and bring meaning to the experience, and not be tempted to hasten the outcome.

Cathartic interventions are *not* concerned with:

- Obtaining information from a client before he or she is ready to disclose;
- Interrupting a client's emotional discharge before it has been completed;
- Encouraging undirected and uncontrolled emotional release, which can be destructive to individuals and/or property;
- Putting clients under pressure to experience an emotional release.

Catalytic Interventions

Catalytic interventions are those that enable the client to develop through a process of self-directed learning and discovery. The aim is to enhance the client's self-awareness and capacity for problem solving. Thus, it is suggested that such interventions are instrumental in the facilitation of individuals to learn about their lives and their living (Heron, 1990). They are enabling and empowering interventions, aiding clients to explore how they could alter patterns in their lives that are counter-productive. They also encourage clients to develop an enquiring approach to living and not to accept self-destructive behaviours at face value, but to identify where the problems may lie and attempt to resolve these through some level of change in their own lives.

Catalytic interventions include:

- Eliciting information by using open ended questions, reflection and paraphrasing;
- Encouraging exploration by the client of his or her present situation and the possible future options;
- Indicating acceptance of the client and how they feel, although not any of the counter-productive behaviour they may exhibit.

Catalytic interventions are *not* concerned with:

- Encouraging the client to work on problems that are assumed by the health care worker;
- Eliciting material to satisfy the curiosity of the health care worker;
- Imposing meanings, prescriptions or interpretations upon the client's material that have not come from the client;
- Encouraging continued client disclosure without responding to or working on that material.

Exercise 10.3: Sustaining Interactions

- *Outcomes*
  Practise listening to the latent content (see Chapter 8 for an explanation of this concept) of a person's speech;
  Practise the use of catalytic and cathartic interventions as means of sustaining interactions;
  Explore and share thoughts and feelings about the use of these skills to sustain interactions.
- *Configuration*
  Pairs.

- *Time*
  Thirty minutes.
- *Materials*
  None.
- *Process*
  Participants each find a partner with whom they have not pre-
  viously worked during this workshop. Each pair identifies a
  speaker and sustainer.
  The speaker identifies a problem that he or she or a client is
  facing and begins to talk about it.
  Using active listening skills (see Chapter 8 for identification of
  these skills), the sustainer identifies the latent content of the
  speaker's words, especially where there are difficult underlying
  feelings associated with the problem.
  The sustainer uses cathartic and/or catalytic interventions (as
  described above) in order to explore the emotional content of the
  speaker's words, while enabling the interaction to continue.
  After 10 minutes, the roles are reversed and the exercise re-
  commences.

Exercise 10.4: Wind Down – Head Roll

- *Outcomes*
  Enable participants to disengage from the previous exercise;
  Reaffirm trust between partners working in pairs;
  Facilitate relaxation.
- *Configuration*
  The same pairs as for the previous exercise.
- *Time*
  Ten minutes.
- *Materials*
  None.
- *Process*
  Working with the same partner as in the previous exercise, each
  pair decides who will wind down first.
  The person who is to wind down first lies on the floor with closed
  eyes, and attempts to relax.
  The supporter kneels behind the partner and cradles the partner's
  head in his or her hands. (Both may find it more comfortable to
  rest the cradled head on the kneeling person's knees.)
  The supporter then *slowly* turns his or her partner's head from
  the left to the right and back, while that person allows the neck
  muscles to relax and be fully supported while using slow and
  small movements.

As the confidence of both participants increases, allow longer but *slow* rolling movements of the neck from left to right.
After three minutes, change roles and repeat the exercise.

NB: Advise participants not to drop their partner's head; it is painful and defeats the object of recreating trust and disengagement!

Plenary Discussion of Exercise 10.3

- *Outcomes*
  Share thoughts and feelings about how word choice can influence the emotional tone of an interaction;
  Share thoughts and feelings about how nonverbal signals can influence the emotional tone of an interaction.

- *Configuration*
  The whole group.

- *Time*
  Approximately 30 minutes.

- *Process*
  The whole group reconvenes to discuss how the emotional content of an interaction can be affected by word choice and nonverbal signals.
  The facilitator encourages a discussion of:
  Whether participants were able to be sensitive to affectively charged words and phrases (examples may be helpful).
  What techniques were helpful in enabling an exploration of sensitive or emotionally charged issues?
  What hindered the catharsis of these emotions?
  In what way were catalytic interventions helpful in sustaining the interaction?

Exercise 10.5: End Game – Stroking

- *Outcomes*
  Enable feedback about each other's performance;
  Reaffirm trust between partners;
  End the section of the workshop on sustaining interactions.

- *Configuration*
  Pairs and the whole group.

- *Time*
  Five minutes.

- *Materials*
  None.

- *Process*
  The whole group sits in a circle.
  Each person is asked to reflect upon the previous exercises, how they personally related to their partners, and one particular thing that they liked or enjoyed about the people with whom they worked.
  Each person is asked to say something positive about his or her partner, with emphasis on the need for honesty and positiveness; concrete examples are encouraged.
  If necessary, the facilitator commences, to set an example.

Theory Input: Talk-Over

- *Outcomes*
  Examine the meaning of 'turn-taking' in interactions and the cues that signal its occurrence;
  Identify the skills associated with encouraging turn-taking to occur;
  Identify the technique of 'talk-over' to help to control an interaction.
- *Configuration*
  The whole group.
- *Time*
  Approximately 20 minutes.
- *Materials*
  Handout of Table 10.5.
- *Process*
  Turn-taking is a natural and necessary part of communication (Trower *et al.* 1978). It refers to the reciprocity that occurs during any interaction in which the participants respect and value each other. There are a number of nonverbal signals that indicate a turn-taking event (e.g. eye contact, tone of voice (particularly at the end of sentences), use of hand/arm signals, posture changes (Dickson *et al.* 1989)), as well as verbal cues. There may be a variety of reasons why a client (or health care worker) might not allow turn-taking to occur, for example:
  Excessive anxiety;
  Preoccupation with internal or external issues (e.g. pain, disturbed family relationships, experiencing hallucinations);
  Conscious or unconscious avoidance of difficult internal or external issues;
  Misperception of turn-taking cues from a partner.

All of these can prevent effective two-way communication and thus preclude any meaningful or therapeutic interaction. In this situation, a health care worker may decide to address this issue with the client. Very occasionally the situation may be so out of control that the client is talking incessantly and preventing any therapeutic communication from taking place. At this point, the health care worker may need to control the interaction to the extent of stopping the client altogether as a prelude to re-establishing reciprocal (two-way) communication. On these occasions the technique of talk-over may be employed.

Give the handout (Table 10.5) to all participants.

Table 10.5 Notes on talk-over

Talk-over is the use of a single word or phrase repeated again and again, if necessary talking across the client, until the individual can no longer persist with his or her own conversation, but is forced to stop and listen to you.

To use the technique effectively the following are suggested:

1. Choose a word or phrase to gain the client's attention. It should be an expression that is significant to the client and has enough impact to capture the client's attention (the client's name is often the best).
2. Begin by saying the word or phrase once, raising your voice slightly, then pause. This is in the hope of catching the person's attention at the outset.
3. If the client does not stop, repeat the key word again and again.
4. *Drop the pitch* of your voice to prevent yourself from simply ending up shouting. Keep the *volume* of your voice only slightly above normal, but again, to prevent a shouting match from developing, do not vary the volume.
5. Keep on repeating the word or phrase, slightly increasing the *tempo* of the repetitions if the client does not stop.
6. Use touch if appropriate, but beware of clients who may reject touch, with the potential for verbal or physical aggression, when in an aroused state.
7. Try to gain eye contact and maintain it.
8. When the client stops talking, immediately use a phrase or sentence that indicates that you are willing to listen to the client but that they need to slow down and address one idea at a time. It is as well to have this phrase ready to use or the client may simply restart speaking rapidly.
9. Once you have regained control, focus on whatever you were most easily able to comprehend. Use an open focused question to pursue this issue, reminding the client to speak slowly.
10. Be prepared to repeat the technique if the client appears to be losing control again. Remind the client that, to help them, you need them to speak slowly. It is not usually so difficult to stop them the second time.

Demonstration

The facilitator(s) demonstrate the skill of talk-over.

Exercise 10.6: Warm Up – Verbal Boxing

- *Outcomes*
  Sensitize participants to the experience of being talked at;
  Enable participants to practise talking at someone;
  Re-engage participants in skills activities;
  Have fun.
- *Configuration*
  Pairs.
- *Time*
  Ten minutes.
- *Materials*
  None.
- *Process*
  Ask the group to divide into pairs.
  The first pair stand face to face in the middle of the group, with the others sitting in a circle around them.
  At a given signal, the pair start to talk at each other on any topic, for 30 seconds, with the intention of preventing each other from talking. Physical touching, screaming and verbal abuse are not allowed.
  The winner is the first person to falter seriously or to cease talking. In the event of an undecided bout, the rest of the group identifies the winner, based upon who spoke the most while ignoring the other person's speech.
  Change pairs and continue until everyone has had a turn.

Exercise 10.7: Role Play – Practising Talk-Over

- *Outcomes*
  Enable participants to practise the skill of talk-over;
  Share thoughts and feelings about the use of the skill of talk-over.
- *Configuration*
  Pairs.
- *Time*
  Approximately 45 minutes, depending on the size of the group.
- *Materials*
  Role play briefing sheets:

  <u>Talk-over role profile (talker)</u> You have just been admitted to a hospital ward and you are anxious about what may happen to you. In fact, you feel very unsure about why you are in hospital. You have a number of worries about your house, your pet, which

is still at home, whether your family knows where you are, and what might happen to you in the future. A health care worker approaches you to ask you some questions.

During the interaction, express as many of the worries as you can. Keep up a steady stream of words. It is vital that you get through to the health care worker how apprehensive you are. Avoid letting the health care worker talk to you. Only stop if you are really compelled by what the health care worker is saying or doing.

Talk-over role profile (controller) You are a health care worker on a hospital ward and you have been asked to see a newly admitted client. You know nothing about this person but you want to ensure that they are able to settle into the ward as easily and comfortably as possible.

During the interaction with the client attempt to use appropriate skills to sustain and control the interaction as necessary. Try to deal with any anxieties the client may express.

Optional: video camera, video tape recorder and television.

- *Process*
  The group divides into pairs. One of each pair chooses to be the 'talker' and the other the 'controller'.
  The talker and the controller are both supplied with role profiles (above); they are allowed a few minutes to get into the role.
  When both partners are ready, they begin, with the controller attempting to control the flow of speech of the talker.
  After three minutes, the role play ceases and the exercise is repeated with the roles reversed.

NB: Video recording of talk-over practice can be very useful and is strongly recommended. However, with large groups it can be time consuming to film all the pairs. In this case, volunteers may be prepared to have their work filmed for use in the discussion.

Exercise 10.8: De-role

- *Outcomes*
  Help workshop participants to distance themselves from the role they were playing;
  Enable participants to relocate back into the workshop.
- *Configuration*
  The whole group.
- *Time*
  Five minutes.

- *Materials*
  None.
- *Process*
  All group members stand in a circle with their arms around each other's waists or holding each other's hands.
  Each member of the group states that they are not the person in the role they have just played, and states their real name, where they are right now and something they are really going to do after the session.

  NB: It is important that everyone who took part in the role play should de-role before the plenary discussion of Example 10.7.

Plenary Discussion of Exercise 10.7

- *Outcomes*
  Identify thoughts and feelings evoked by having to talk over a client and take control;
  Share thoughts and feelings about having to control an interaction;
  Share thoughts and feelings about deciding when to 'let go' of the control you have taken.
- *Configuration*
  The whole group.
- *Time*
  Approximately 30 minutes.
- *Process*
  The whole group reconvenes to discuss the issues raised by having to take control of a conversation.
  The facilitator needs to encourage a discussion of:
     Thoughts and feelings about controlling and being controlled in an interaction;
     Various aspects of the technique of talk-over;
     The ease and/or difficulty of its use;
     Its merit as a tool within a health worker–client relationship.
  The reading list at the end of this chapter can be distributed at this point.

Exercise 10.8: Evaluation of the Workshop

- *Outcomes*
  Help workshop participants to identify what they liked most and least about the workshop as a whole;

Enable facilitators to identify parts of the workshop that might need alteration in the future;
Allow time for reflection upon practice and skills acquisition.

- *Configuration*
  The whole group.
- *Time*
  Fifteen minutes.
- *Process*
  The whole group sits in a circle.
  Each member of the group in turn states one thing about the workshop that they would like to change. This can include the material, the exercises or their own performance during the day. Members may 'pass' at their turn, but must not justify or respond to requests for justification of any statement they make.
  After each member has responded or 'passed', then each member in turn states one thing they feel they have achieved during the course of the workshop.

Reading List

Heron, J. (1990) *Helping the Client – a Creative Practical Guide*. Sage, London.

Nelson-Jones, R. (1990) *Human Relationship Skills*. Cassell, London, Chapter 5.

Porritt, L. (1990) *Interaction Strategies – an Introduction for Health Professionals*. Churchill Livingstone, Melbourne, Chapter 6.

Trower, P., Bryant, B. and Argyle, M. (1978) *Social Skills and Mental Health*. Methuen, London.

Chapter 11

Closing Interactions

In Chapter 9 we discussed the importance of opening interactions to the development of relationships with clients. However, of equal importance in working with clients is the way in which therapeutic interactions are concluded and how the final closure of a relationship takes place (Culley, 1991). With the pressure on health care workers to get through more work with clients in a shorter space of time, shorter meetings with clients, or the failure to take time over the way client–worker relationships are concluded, may be a temptation. However, if the conclusion of a meeting or the client–worker relationship is perceived as unsatisfactory by the client, this could result in difficulties in maintaining or developing subsequent therapeutic relationships with that person. It is, therefore, essential to examine various aspects of closing interactions, ensuring that this is done as constructively as possible.

This workshop is aimed at exploring the effective use of closing strategies when interacting with clients. In considering endings, it is necessary to identify whether or not it is only the immediate exchange that is ending or the relationship as a whole. This workshop will examine different approaches to effectively facilitate either type of ending. It must be stressed, however, that when a health care worker–client relationship is ending, it is crucial that the work takes place over an extended period. This is to enable a discussion of the pending separation between the client and health care worker and its meaning for both people, and to offer an opportunity for each individual to raise issues that might otherwise have been left unacknowledged. As a result, the relationship can be brought to a more satisfactory close, although it is still possible that some of the issues may remain unresolved. It is, therefore, important that health care workers should become aware of strategies to close interactions that will promote a satisfactory ending and, ultimately, client satisfaction.

Learning Outcomes

1. Identify the importance of closing an interaction effectively;
2. Recall the verbal and nonverbal elements of closing interactions;
3. Differentiate between closing each interaction and overall endings;
4. Explore the closing strategies identified by Saunders (1986);
5. Examine the effect that ending interactions may have on the health care worker–client relationship;
6. Experience when an interaction is inappropriately discontinued;
7. Share thoughts and feelings about adequate and inadequate endings.

Introduction to the Workshop

The facilitators need to state:

- *Learning outcomes for the workshop*
- *Methods used* Identify the teaching/learning methods to be used, suggesting that full participation will greatly enhance the learning outcomes, especially with the use of video recording equipment. Also obtain agreement from participants that personal material divulged during the workshop will not be disclosed outside the group.
- *Time considerations* Make explicit the overall time for the workshop, and the time taken for breaks and when these might occur. Negotiate some flexibility in timing (up to 15 minutes either side of a stated time) but ensure that you finish on time.
- *Housekeeping issues* Locations of other rooms, toilet facilities, and eating and drinking arrangements; rules about smoking (e.g. designated areas, although we advise not to allow smoking during the workshop); issues concerning participants' safety, including fire procedures and those relating to personal items such as clothing, jewellery and footwear.

Theory Input: Closing Interactions

- *Outcomes*
  Describe the theoretical framework for closing interactions proposed by Saunders (1986);

Examine the possible use of different types of intervention when closing interactions;
Examine the meanings underpinning the concept of closing interactions.

- *Configuration*
  The whole group.
- *Time*
  Approximately 20 minutes.
- *Materials*
  Handout of the four closing formats, with subtypes (Saunders, 1986):
  1. Factual: summary, initiating or inviting questions, developing future links;
  2. Motivational: explicitly motivating statements, thought-provoking comments, future orientation statements;
  3. Social: concluding task-related statements, nontask-related statements, acknowledgement statements;
  4. Perceptual: final verbal closure markers, nonverbal closure markers.
- *Process*
  Before the theory input begins, distribute the handout to the group.

Introduction

The ending of an interaction and a relationship is as important as its beginning. One change experienced in the relationship is decreased access, potentially resulting in a sense of sadness and loss for both people (Franchino, 1989). However, to counteract a sudden cessation of contact, a variety of rituals have been developed by humans to signify this end, such as changes in posture, voice tone, pauses and types of words used (Goffman, 1972). Schegloff and Sacks (1973) have suggested that these signals are used so that both interactors can conclude that the contact will end unambiguously, thus terminating the interaction. Although passing encounters do not usually result in full ending rituals, these formalities are important at other times to confirm that there will no longer be contact or that contact will be suspended for a time.

Ending an interaction effectively performs a number of functions. If there is planned future contact, it can increase anticipation of the next encounter. There can be a review of what has taken place and the scene set for the next meeting. Also, goals and actions to be accomplished by the next session may be identified. Final endings can help the participants to acknowledge that no further contact will take place, seeing this both as a sad time and one that presents a challenge for future action. Whichever type of ending is being experienced, the skills used will depend upon a number of factors, such as the individual's personal experiences, cultural background, social position, intellect and other characteristics.

Having given an indication of some of the purposes of ending interactions, the question of its meaning now arises. Saunders (1986) has proposed that it is:

> ...directing attention to the termination of social exchange by summarising the main issues which have been discussed, drawing attention to what will happen in the future, and finally, breaking interpersonal contact without making participants feel rejected or shunned (p. 190).

She suggests that there are four different forms to be used when closing interactions, which are subsequently divided into subtypes. These closing strategies may be employed to increase awareness and the choice of how endings may take place with clients. The four closing formats, with subtypes, are outlined briefly in the handout. Below is a more detailed description of each. It must be remembered that more than one of these closing strategies can be used within a single interaction.

Factual Closing

This type of ending strategy is used when future contact is expected and it is desirable to clarify the emotional and cognitive aspects of the interaction. An attempt is made to link the present discussions with the client's potential future. Here, attention is given to *primacy* and *recency* effects; the beginning and end of an interaction are more likely to be remembered than the middle (Gregg, 1986). Below are the subcategories of this type of closing strategy.

Summary

In this type of ending, the health care worker offers a summary of the session from his or her understanding. It is used to reiterate the main points that have been covered and affords time to clarify any misunderstandings. The value of this is to ensure that information concerning any work to be undertaken between meetings is accurate and agreed. A summary also helps the client to assess his or her development, offering a clearer indication of the overall progress. The process of summing up at regular intervals within a meeting helps the retention of information, especially if there has been a great deal within the session. The final summary then serves as a reinforcement for the retention of this material.

Initiating or Inviting Questions

This involves asking specific questions in order to check the accuracy of what has been understood, and to evaluate, with the client, what benefit has been derived from the discussions. It also affords an opportunity to open up the ending for questions by the client, reducing the risk that he or she will leave with unvoiced concerns. Asking and inviting questions can also help to consolidate the learning that has taken place.

Developing Future Links

This type of ending is aimed at raising awareness of the work that will continue in future sessions. It looks ahead at tasks and decisions that require further attention. It also helps to identify concerns that the client may have about this future work. Thus, there is ultimately a large element of support offered by the health care worker when using this type of closing strategy.

Motivational Closing

Motivational endings are used to help to mobilize individuals into action. They help to concretize what has happened thus far and to consider how to use ideas being developed by the client. They encourage clients to reflect upon issues identified in discussions, explore various permutations, and merge the results with earlier ideas. When using these approaches to close interactions, it is possible to establish a schedule for future work and identify any required action. This type of ending tends to be used when future meetings are planned and when it is counter-productive to leave the client with a perception of finality.

Explicitly Motivating Statements

These are specific statements that encourage the elicitation of explicit actions from clients in order to help them to move towards a solution to their difficulties. They help clients to verbalize and clarify these actions. These can be statements such as, 'You said that you would like to . . .', or 'I believe that it *would* be wise for you to take [that] action', or questions such as, 'What do you think is the best way to deal with . . .?'

Thought-Provoking Comments

This type of closure creates a connection between the present experiences of the client and what is anticipated for the future. It often leaves the client with more questions than answers, encouraging reflection upon what action might be taken after the session. An example of this type of closure might be, 'If . . . happens, what do you imagine you might . . . [say, think, do, etc.].'

Future Orientation Statements

Using this type of closure actively encourages the client to explore (once the session is finished) the material that has been internalized and how it may be used in new situations. It is an explicit encouragement to do 'homework' between sessions, with the understanding that feedback about this homework will occur at the start of the next session. The future orientation of this closure attempts to help the client to recognize the value of his or her exploratory work.

Social Closing

Social closure strategies can be used in both a final ending and when there is planned future contact. They aim to maintain the relationship through the period without communication and encourage the client to 'look forward' to the next discussion. If it is the last meeting, they aim to provide a 'good' ending, which is positively rewarding for the client and the health care worker. Using this type of closing strategy can also establish whether or not the interaction has been of benefit to the client. It offers an opportunity to identify feelings, good or bad, that may be left at the end of the encounter.

Concluding Task-Related Statements

This ending strategy offers a social reward to the client for achievements. It takes account of what has been accomplished, acknowledging its worth for the client. In doing this, it also serves as a supportive intervention.

Nontask-Related Statements

Using this type of ending effectively depends upon the situation and the relationship between the client and the health care worker. It can be used to lighten the ending to a difficult session or to acknowledge that the relationship has not been damaged as a result of difficulties in the session. It always takes the form of a friendly, warm, and genuine use of either a statement or a question that is nonwork related, for example, 'Take care now', or 'Hope you enjoy your holiday.'

Acknowledgement Statements

These acknowledge a value that the health care worker places on discussions with the client. They are often used as a clear message signalling the completion of the interaction and recognizing its worth. It is important that these statements are used in an atmosphere of genuine acceptance of the client. Such expressions as, 'I enjoyed our discussions', or 'I look forward to our next meeting', are examples of this type of closure strategy.

Perceptual Closing

This type of ending aims to ensure that there is no ambiguity between the health care worker and the client that the interaction is ending. It provides such cues as gestures and body posture, which indicate an end to the interaction and that it is time to part company. Schegloff and Sacks (1973) suggest that many nonverbal signals, such as changes in distance, posture and gaze, accompany verbal utterances to emphasize such an ending. It is important to combine verbal and nonverbal cues when closing an interaction, to ensure that the participants are clear that there will be no further contact.

Final Verbal Closure Markers

These constitute the verbal aspects of closure. They are the words used to delineate whether or not the parting is final or will be followed up. The form the words can take depends upon the relationship. The words used can also have an effect upon whether or not it is a 'good' parting and can affect subsequent meetings. Therefore, being aware when familiar words or formal words need to be used can be beneficial to future meetings. Examples of verbal markers are: 'So long', or 'I'll see you next week', or 'Goodbye.'

Nonverbal Closure Markers

These are the nonverbal aspects of closure that indicate when an encounter is coming to an end. They involve such movements as changing posture (e.g. moving to the edge of your seat, moving further away from the other person, breaking eye contact, arm/hand movements). Again, depending upon the relationship, other closure markers may be employed, such as a handshake or a hug, both of which are recognized cross-culturally as signals used to end interactions.

Exercise 11.1: Warm Up – 'The sun shines on anyone who ...'

● *Outcomes*
   Help to prepare participants to take part in the ensuing role play exercises;
   Increase group cohesion;
   Have fun.

● *Configuration*
   The whole group.

● *Time*
   Five minutes.

● *Materials*
   None.

● *Process*
   The whole group sits in a circle; there is one chair less than the number of participants.
   One of the participants stands in the centre of the circle.
   He or she then makes the statement: 'The sun shines on anyone who ...', finishing the sentence with the name of a piece of clothing, its colour, a place they may have been, something seen on television or in the cinema etc., for example, 'The sun shines on anyone who has brown shoes.'
   Those participants who's experience, appearance, etc. corresponds to what has been said, have to change chairs.
   The person in the centre tries at this time to sit on one of the recently vacated chairs.
   If successful, a new individual will be in the centre and he or she will make the statement: 'The sun shines on anyone who ...', but he or she repeats the statement with a different ending.
   The whole process is repeated for no more than five minutes.

Exercise 11.2: Ending Motto

- *Outcomes*
  Focus participants' thinking towards closing interactions;
  Help participants to begin to identify the importance of endings;
  Have fun.
- *Configuration*
  Individuals, who then make pairs, then make fours, etc. until all participants become a single group.
- *Time*
  Up to 30 minutes: five minutes for each part and 10 minutes for a short discussion.
- *Materials*
  Paper and pens.
- *Process*
  Individually, each participant writes a motto, which represents what endings mean to them.
  They then join a partner and the pair make up a joint motto about what endings mean, using the ones they have written as individuals.
  Then that pair joins with another pair to make up another composite motto about the meaning of endings.
  This procedure continues until the final motto represents a total group effort.
  After the final motto has been presented, the group discusses, for about 10 minutes, the following: the process of working co-operatively; and the feelings involved in thinking and discussing endings.

Exercise 11.3: Ending Interactions

- *Outcomes*
  Increase the participants' awareness of the importance of ending an interaction effectively;
  Experience the thoughts and feelings associated with ending an interaction, both when there are subsequent sessions and as a final session;
  Practise using the different endings identified by Saunders (1986);
  Practise time management;
  Share thoughts and feelings about closing interactions when the therapeutic relationship will continue and also when it will end.
- *Configuration*
  Small groups of three or possibly four (but no more).

- *Time*
  Total 50 minutes: 15 minutes for each person in the role; five minutes feedback from the observer and client after *each* session; 10 minutes for the small group to have an overall discussion.

- *Materials*
  Observer sheets, with space for writing underneath the following instructions:

  Please write down the verbal and nonverbal behaviour that you think is important to feed back to the listener during the skills practice discussion, especially in relation to closing the interaction. Also please note, for discussion, the category of closure, from those identified by Saunders (1986), that has been used.

- *Process*
  In triads, identify who will be: the health care worker; the client; and the observer(s).

  The client and the health care worker talk for 15 minutes about something important to the client.

  The health care worker makes it explicit to the client, in a warm, caring manner, that the discussion can be only for 15 minutes.

  It is the health care worker's responsibility to ensure that the interaction is closed therapeutically in the time allowed.

  After the first 15 minutes of the exercise, the health care worker in each group has a five-minute feedback from the observer and the client on his or her performance.

  Repeat the exercise, with a different speaker, listener and observer each time.

  The first health care worker in the triad responds as though they will be seeing the client on subsequent occasions.

  The second health care worker in the triad responds to the client as though this is the last meeting they will have.

  The observer fills in the observer sheet (above), writing about how they perceived the health care worker closed the interaction, giving feedback to the health care worker for about five minutes after each session.

  The triads have an overall discussion of the exercise for 10 minutes, after two people have been in the health care worker role.

Exercise 11.4: De-role

- *Outcomes*
  Help participants to distance themselves from the role they were playing;

Help participants to re-engage with the group as themselves rather than from within the role they have just played.

- *Configuration*
  All participants in a role from the previous exercise.
- *Time*
  Five minutes.
- *Materials*
  None.
- *Process*
  All participants in the previous exercise stand in a circle with their arms around each other's waists.

  Each person in turn states that they are not the person in the role they have just played, and states their real name, where they are right now, and something that is true about them at that moment (e.g. what they are wearing, how they are feeling or what they are doing).

NB: It is important that everyone who took part in the role play should de-role before the plenary discussion of Exercise 11.3.

Plenary Discussion of Exercise 11.3

- *Outcomes*
  Identify thoughts and feelings associated with closing interactions in two circumstances: when the relationship will continue and when the relationship is finally ending;
  Discuss time management in relation to ending sessions.
- *Configuration*
  The whole group.
- *Time*
  Approximately 20 minutes.
- *Process*
  The whole group sits in a circle.
  A discussion is facilitated about feelings associated with being in either the health care worker's or the client's role.

Exercise 11.5: Nonending Role Play

- *Outcomes*
  Experience, as the client, the thoughts and feelings associated with having an interaction end unsatisfactorily;
  Experience, as the health care worker, the thoughts and feelings associated with ending an interaction unsatisfactorily.

- *Configuration*
  Pairs.
- *Time*
  Ten minutes.
- *Materials*
  None.
- *Process*
  NB: *Do not introduce the exercise by its title.*
  The group divides into pairs (a facilitator may need to join in one group or one group may need to be in a three, with one person as the observer).
  Identify one person as the health care worker and one as the client.
  The facilitators take the health care workers out of room before the exercise begins to tell them that they must break the discussion off abruptly after 10 minutes, but they are not to let the speaker know that this will happen, either verbally or nonverbally.
  It is important that the interaction should relate to a relatively light-hearted work problem.
  The health care worker encourages the client to talk openly.
  After 10 minutes, the health care worker abruptly breaks off the discussion (e.g. by stopping talking, altering the topic completely, looking away and not responding, getting up and walking away, etc.).

Exercise 11.6: De-role

- *Outcomes*
  Enable participants to distance themselves from the role they were playing;
  Help participants to re-engage with the group as themselves rather than from within the role they have just played.
- *Configuration*
  All participants in a role from the previous exercise.
- *Time*
  Five minutes.
- *Materials*
  None.
- *Process*
  All participants in the previous exercise stand in a circle with their arms around each other's waists.
  Each person in turn states that they are not the person in the

role they have just played, and states their real name, where they are right now, and something that is true about them at that moment (e.g. what they are wearing, how they are feeling or what they are doing).

NB: It is *very* important that everyone who took part in the roleplay should de-role before the plenary discussion of Exercise 11.5.

Plenary Discussion of Exercise 11.5

- *Outcomes*
  Share thoughts and feelings about the experience of not having your interaction end satisfactorily;
  Share thoughts and feelings about the experience of ending an interaction abruptly;
  Make comparisons between effective and ineffective endings.
- *Configuration*
  The whole group.
- *Time*
  Approximately 20 minutes.
- *Process*
  The whole group sits in a circle.
  Facilitate a discussion about:
    What constitutes ineffective endings;
    The feelings that ineffective endings engender;
    Possible outcomes for the client and health care worker when an interaction/relationship is ended unsatisfactorily.

Exercise 11.7: Verbal and Nonverbal Components of Effective Closing

- *Outcomes*
  Identify the verbal and nonverbal elements of communication associated with closing an interaction effectively;
  Identify the verbal and nonverbal elements of communication associated with different types of endings.
- *Configuration*
  Initially, the group divides into two, then the whole group joins together.
- *Time*
  Thirty minutes.

- *Materials*
  Flip-chart paper;
  Pens;
  Blu-tac.

- *Process*
  The group divides into two equal groups.
  One group writes down on a large piece of paper the verbal components of effective closing, while the other group writes down the nonverbal components of effective closing.
  After 10 minutes, the groups rejoin, put their papers up on the wall and, for about 20 minutes, discuss what they have written.

Exercise 11.8: Evaluation of the Workshop

- *Outcomes*
  Help the participants to identify what they liked most and liked least about the workshop as a whole;
  Enable the facilitator(s) to identify parts of the workshop that might be altered in the future;
  Allow time for participants to reflect upon the skills acquired and their practice.

- *Configuration*
  The whole group.

- *Time*
  Approximately 15 minutes.

- *Process*
  Each participant, including the facilitator, is asked to say one thing they liked least about the workshop, or 'pass'.
  After all participants have responded, the facilitator asks each person to say one thing they liked most about this workshop, or 'pass'.
  Participants are requested not to give or respond to any request for justification of their statements. They may also decline to give feedback by stating 'No comment', or 'Pass'.
  If used, evaluation forms can be given at this stage.

Reading List

Culley, S. (1991) *Integrative Counselling Skills in Action*. Sage, London.

Dickson, D.A., Hargie, O. and Morrow, N.C. (1989) *Communication Skills Training for Health Professionals*. Chapman and Hall, London.

Franchino, L. (1989) *Bereavement and Counselling*. Counselling Services, Weybridge.

Saunders, C. (1986) Opening and closing. In *Communications Skills*. (ed. O. Hargie) Routledge, London.

Chapter 12

Summary and Afterword

This book has directed the reader in an exploration of some of the theories of competent communications and how they apply in health care settings. The series of structured workshops can be used by teachers and trainers as a foundation for training people who work in health care settings and use communication as a central part of their work with clients. This includes professionally qualified staff, those in training, paid workers and volunteers.

We believe that there is a therapeutic value in open, clear communications with clients and that this should be delivered by competent practitioners who have had the opportunity for their practice to be guided by theory. We hope that a balance has been struck between the theoretical and the practical. We do not suggest that the way we have structured the workshops and the style of facilitation that underpins them are the only ways in which communication skills can be taught. We would certainly recommend that facilitators or trainers using the workshops should consider them as the building blocks from which to develop material relevant to the needs of participants in a style that is acceptable to the trainers. This inevitably means designing modifications in the pursuit of a 'tailored to fit' programme of material. We are clear that adaptation rather than imitation is the sincerest form of flattery.

In this book, we have produced a resource that we hope will enhance knowledge and understanding of the concepts of communication, at the same time providing tools in the form of the workshops and their constituent exercises to help to develop the skills of effective, therapeutic communication. Learning a skill requires both knowledge of the concepts and an opportunity to rehearse and receive feedback about practise of the skills (Lovell, 1982; Minton, 1991; Quinn, 1995). Consequently, we have placed emphasis upon the 'doing' and 'feeling' of communicating as well as upon the 'knowing'. In integrating these within the workshops, we suggest that it may be possible to explore new skills and understanding in the relatively safe 'laboratory' environment of the training venue, prior to incorporating these into work with clients.

Although within the book we identify one specific model to inform our understanding of communication skills (see Chapter 2), this was done principally to provide a rationale for the structure of the workshops. We acknowledge that no one model offers a complete explanation for all of the complexities of communication and that the choice of model may depend upon the purposes of communication as well as the beliefs and values of the communicators. We hope that the adoption of a particular model has helped rather than hindered the reader. We would, therefore, encourage teachers and trainers to consider other approaches that might inform the act of communicating, while at the same time providing a map or structure for the sequencing of the material or workshops that they provide.

In Chapter 3 we place particular emphasis on the concept of psychological safety, suggesting that its absence from interactions between health care worker and client will prevent open and clear communications. In the course of running workshops to train various types of health care workers, it has become clear to us that psychological safety is a concept best dealt with by raising the awareness of the participants' own needs for safety within the training sessions and acting as role models for the provision of this safety. We have emphasized the need to prepare participants for the work they will be undertaking and not to compel them to take part in exercises or teaching techniques for which they are not yet ready. In particular, the use of video equipment can raise anxiety and we make no apologies for the importance attached to preparing them for this work. Although participants may have obligations of their own (to learn new skills in order to do their job and to encourage and support the learning of fellow participants within the group), allowing them some control over the pace of their own learning will give a very clear message about the empathy and respect that is their right. From this will stem an appreciation of the rights of their clients to similar treatment.

The educational strategy behind all of these workshops is that of experiential teaching, which we believe to be the most appropriate and effective method to teach communication skills. This is a belief supported by others working in this field (Burnard, 1989b, 1990; Egan, 1990b; Kagan et al. 1986; McKay et al. 1983; Pfeiffer, 1985). Chapter 4 gave a selected review of the rationale behind the use of experiential teaching, and, as with earlier chapters, while not exhaustive, it directs readers to other texts and sources. One of the central tenets of experiential training is that people learn by doing; we are clear that learning to communicate effectively with clients cannot be learned without doing and discovering. Consequently, the workshops contain numerous large and small group exercises, which enable the participants to practise what they learn. Although we have presented specific examples and case vignettes for some of those exercises, facilitators running their own workshops based upon this book may find it worthwhile to produce examples drawn from their own experiences or those of the participants with whom they are working. This form of co-operation will not only provide constructive examples but will also demonstrate the collaborative nature of the learning process and the respect and regard that is so vital to the communication process between individuals. It will also help to reduce the often unconscious power differential that exists between instructor and participant in more traditional forms of teaching and provide a model for practice where participants feel secure enough to bridge the inequality of power frequently inherent in relationships between clients and health care workers.

However, some participants might prefer a more structured approach to learning. Additionally, large numbers undertaking training or the limited availability of resources may necessitate a more inductive approach. For this reason we have attempted within each workshop to use both inductive and deductive teaching methods, finding a place for direct information-giving alongside the experiential work. Achieving the right balance between these styles is central to the process of adapting the material, and we suggest that one of the keys to successful communication skills training lies in the blending of these approaches to learning without relying too heavily upon one or the other.

The workshops contained in Part II of this book provide an entire course in communication skills. When used in this way, they will be seen to move from the general to the specific. Thus, in Chapter 5 we offered an overview of the elements of communication, verbal and nonverbal, and the way these are combined in the key skill of active listening. Subsequent chapters covered each of these elements in more detail. The last three chapters of the book have presented workshops designed to increase not only the breadth of learning communication skills but also its depth by addressing stages that are present in most interpersonal communications. Chapter 9 examined the skills of opening interactions, while Chapter 10 covered sustaining and controlling interactions, acknowledging that interactions may need to be sustained, especially when there is some degree of reticence on the part of the client. Alternatively, there may be rare occasions when it is necessary to exert some control on the interaction, slowing the pace or stopping it to alter the direction, thus enabling the client and health care worker to achieve a greater degree of mutuality.

The final chapter explored the ending of interactions. This is an aspect of communication that has not received a great deal of attention (exceptions can be found in Culley (1991) and Franchino (1989)). It was appropriate that the last workshop of the book should address this potentially emotive subject, because it is not just about ending an interaction, but also about ending a genuine, helping relationship with all of the emotional inference that this brings. Thus, the exercises and the discussions in this workshop aimed to look at both aspects of endings, temporary, as in the ending of a session within a series of sessions, or the ending of the relationship in total. This chapter on closing interactions seemed a fitting ending to the series of workshops.

In our experience of running these workshops, by the time the participants have come to the end, they have altered radically the way in which they view the process of communicating with clients. Previous comments about communicating being a natural process governed only by experience and common sense have been replaced, in the main, by a sense of discovery at the complexity and depth of meaning that can be attached to apparently mundane interactions. Participants seem to grow in confidence as they discover their own abilities in using the skills they have learned when working with clients. These skills have also given a greater dimension to their understanding and insight into their clients and they take from the workshops an eagerness to continue this learning process. We believe that, regardless of how skilled practitioners are in communicating, there is always a need to improve. We suggest to anyone considering offering communication skills training that they should be aware of the continuing needs of health care workers to maintain, refine and develop their skills beyond what is offered in these workshops.

Continuing training or support does not have to be elaborate or costly. It will enable those who have begun the process of learning to enhance their skills and to feel valued as they do so. Additional training may include 'top up' or review sessions held some months after the end of the workshops. It might also involve organizing ongoing peer group support meetings in which problems of communication with clients can be discussed. In some situations, it may be possible for more experienced staff to be paired with newer staff to provide regular, formal supervision or mentorship.

We regularly see press reports with headlines such as, 'The Health Service Ombudsman has highlighted poor communication as one of the main causes of breakdown in services to NHS patients' (*Nursing Standard*, 1995: p. 10). These indicate the extent to which incomplete communication and mixed messages lead to breakdowns not only in relations between clients and health care workers but also between workers and managers. If, as suggested in Chapter 1, we not only 'say what we mean' but also 'mean what we say', poor communication would be less likely to occur. To mean what we say and say what we mean requires conscious, thoughtful decisions and actions taken by competent, confident people. We hope that those who have used this book will have helped others to become, or have themselves become, more competent and facilitative when communicating with clients and their carers.

Exercise Source Books

The books listed below are included to increase the reader's choices when using experiential techniques and to supplement the exercises found in this book. We would also like to acknowledge that some of the exercises that have been used in this book are adaptations from some of these source books.

Bond, M. and Kilty, J. (1982) *Practical Methods of Dealing with Stress.* (Human Potential Research Project.) University of Surrey, Guildford.

Brandes, D. and Phillips, H. (1977) *Gamesters' Handbook.* Hutchinson, London.

Brandes, D. (1982) *Gamesters' Handbook Two.* Hutchinson, London.

Burnard, P. (1989) *Teaching Interpersonal Skills: A Handbook of Experiential Learning for Health Professionals.* Chapman & Hall, London.

Burnard, P. (1990) *Learning Human Skills: A Guide for Nurses*, 2nd ed. Heinemann Nursing, London.

Egan, G. (1990) *Exercises in Helping Skills: A Training Manual to Accompany The Skilled Helper.* Brooks/Cole, Pacific Grove, CA.

Franchino, L. (1989) *Bereavement and Counselling.* Counselling Services, Weybridge.

Jelfs, M. (1982) *Manual for Action.* Action Resources Group, London.

Jennings, S. (1986) *Creative Drama in Groupwork.* Winslow Press, Oxford.

Kagan, C., Evans, J. and Kay, B. (1986) *A Manual of Interpersonal Skills for Nurses: An Experimental Approach.* Harper & Row, London.

Kirby, A. (1992) *Games for Trainers (Vol. 1).* Gower, Aldershot.

Kirby, A. (1992) *Games for Trainers (Vol. 2).* Gower, Aldershot.

Lewis, H.R. and Streitfeld, H.S. (1970) *Growth Games.* ABACUS, London.

McKay, M., Davis, M. and Fanning, P. (1983) *Messages: The Communication Skills Book.* New Harbinger, Oakland, CA.

Nelson-Jones R. (1990) *Human Relationship Skills.* Cassell Educational, London.

Pfeiffer, J.W. and Jones, J.J. (1969–1985) *A Handbook of Structured Experiences for Human Relations Training, Vol. I–X.* University Associates Publishers and Consultants, San Diego, CA.

Priestly, P., McGuire, J., Flegg, D., Hemsley, V. and Welham, D. (1978) *Social Skills and Personal Problem Solving: A Handbook of Methods.* Tavistock, London.

Remocker, A.J. and Storch, E.T. (1987) *Action Speaks Louder: A Handbook of Structured Group Techniques*, 4th ed. Churchill Livingstone, Edinburgh.

Townend, A. (1985) *Assertion Training.* FPA Education Unit, London.

Trower, P., Bryant, B. and Argyle, M. (1978) *Social Skills and Mental Health.* Methuen, London.

References

Argyle, M. (1983) *The Psychology of Interpersonal Behaviour*, 4th ed. Penguin, Harmondsworth.

Argyle, M. (1988) *Bodily Communication*, 2nd ed. Routledge, London.

Arnetz, B.B., Wasserman, J., Petrini, B., Brenner, S.O., Levi, L., Eneroth, P., Salovaara, H., Hjelm., R., Salovaara, L., Theorell, T. and Petterson, I.L. (1987) Immune function in unemployed women. *Psychosomatic Medicine* **49**, 3–12.

Ausubel, D. (1984) Learning as constructed meaning. In *New Directions in Educational Psychology: 1. Learning and Teaching*. (ed. N. Entwistle) Falmer, London, p. 71.

Bailey, K.G. and Sowder, W.J. (1970) Audiotape and videotape self confrontation in psychotherapy. *Psychological Bulletin* **74**, 127–37.

Bandura, A. (1977) *Social Learning Theory*. Prentice Hall, Englewood Cliffs, NJ.

Barber, P. (1988) *Applied Cognitive Psychology*. Routledge, London.

Beck, C.M., Rawlins, R.P. and Williams, S.R. (1988) *Mental Health – Psychiatric Nursing: A Holistic Life-cycle Approach*, 2nd ed. Mosby, St Louis, MO.

Berger, C.R. (1988) Uncertainty and information exchange in developing relationships. In *Handbook of Personal Relationships: theory, research, and interventions*. (ed. S. Duck) Wiley, Chichester Chapter,13.

Birdwhistell, R. (1970) *Kinesics and Context*. University of Philadelphia Press, Philadelphia, PA.

Bond, M.R. (1971) The relation of pain to the Eysenck Personality Inventory, Cornell Medical Index and the Whitely Index of Hypochondriasis. *British Journal of Psychiatry* **119**, 671–78.

Bowlby, J. (1973) *Attachment and Loss Vol. II: Separation, Anxiety and Anger.* Hogarth Press, London.

Bradley, J.C. and Edinberg, M.A. (1990) *Communication in the Nursing Context*, 3rd ed. Appleton and Lange, Norwalk, CT.

Brown, D. and Pedder, J. (1991) *Introduction to Psychotherapy – an Outline of Psychodynamic Principles and Practice*. Routledge, London.

Brown, G.W. and Harris, T. (1978) *Social Origins of Depression*. Tavistock, London.

Burnard, P. (1989a) Exploring nurse educators' views of experiential learning: a pilot study. *Nurse Education Today* **9**, 39–45.

Burnard, P. (1989b) *Teaching Interpersonal Skills: a Handbook of Experiential Learning for Health Professionals*. Chapman & Hall, London.

Burnard, P. (1990) *Learning Human Skills: A Guide for Nurses*, 2nd ed. Heinemann Nursing, London.

Care Sector Consortium. (1992) *Care Sector Consortium: National Occupational Standards for Care*. City and Guilds of London.

Carroll, L. (1946) *Alice's Adventures in Wonderland*. Puffin, Harmondsworth.

Chomsky, N. (1965) *Aspects on the Theory of Syntax*. MIT Press, Cambridge, MA.

Corney, R., Everett, H., Howells, A. and Crowther, M. (1992) The care of patients undergoing surgery for gynaecological cancer: the need for information, emotional support and counselling. *Journal of Advanced Nursing* **17**, 667–71.

Cromer, R.E. (1991) *Language and Thought in Normal and Handicapped Children*. Basil Blackwell, Cambridge, MA.

Culley, S. (1991) *Integrative Counselling Skills in Action*. Sage, London.

Darbyshire, P. (1993) In defence of pedagogy: a critique of the notion of andragogy. *Nurse Education Today* **13**, 328–35.

Department of Health. (1992) *The Health of the Nation: A Strategy for Health in England*. HMSO, London.

Dickson, D.A., Hargie, O. and Morrow, N.C. (1989) *Communication Skills Training for Health Professionals*. Chapman and Hall, London.

Donaldson, M. (1978) *Children's Minds*. Fontana, London.

Egan, G (1990a) *The Skilled Helper: a Systematic Approach to Effective Helping*, 4th ed. Brooks/Cole, Pacific Grove, CA.

Egan, G. (1990b) *Exercises in Helping Skills: A Training Manual to Accompany The Skilled Helper*. Brooks/Cole, Pacific Grove, CA.

Eimas, P., Siqueland, E.R., Jusczyk, P. and Vigorito, J. (1971) Speech perception in infants. *Science* **171**, 303–6.

Ellis, A. and Beattie, G. (1986) *The Psychology of Language and Communication*. Lawrence Erlbaum, Hove.

Erikson, E.H. (1969) *Childhood and Society*. Penguin, Harmondsworth.

Fielding, R.G. and Llewelyn, S.P. (1987) Communication training in nursing may damage your health and enthusiasm – some warnings. *Journal of Advanced Nursing* **12**, 281–90.

Franchino, L. (1989) *Bereavement and Counselling*. Counselling Services, Weybridge.

Gagne, R. (1985) *The Conditions of Learning and Theory of Instruction*, 4th ed. Holt, Rinehart and Winston, New York.

Garnham, A. (1985) *Psycholinguistics: Central Topics*. Methuen, London, Chapter 3.

Goffman, E. (1971) *Strategic Interactions*. Basil Blackwell, Oxford.

Goffman, E. (1972) *Relations in Public: Micro-studies of the Public Order*. Penguin, Harmondsworth.

Green, J. (1987) *Memory, Thinking, and Language*. Methuen, London.

Gregg, V.H. (1986) *Introduction to Human Memory*. Routledge & Kegan Paul, London.

Griffiths, R.D.P. (1974) Videotape feedback as a therapist technique – retrospect and prospect. *Behaviour Research and Therapy* **12**, 1–8.

Haley, T.J. and Dowd, E.T. (1988) Responses of deaf adolescents to differences in counsellor method of communication and disability status. *Journal of Counselling Psychology* **35**, 258–62.

Hampson, S.E. (1988) *The Construction of Personality*, 2nd ed. Routledge & Kegan Paul, London.

Hardin, S.B. and Halaris, A.L. (1983) Nonverbal communication of patients and high and low empathy nurses. *Journal of Psychosocial Nursing and Mental Health* **21**, 14–20.

Hargie, O., ed. (1986) *A Handbook of Communication Skills*. Routledge, London.

Hayward, J. (1975) *Information – a Prescription Against Pain*. Royal College of Nursing, London.

Henry, J. (1989) Meaning and practice in experiential learning. In *Making Sense of Experiential Learning: Diversity in Theory and Practice*. (eds S. Warner Weil and I. McGill) The Society for Research into Higher Education and Open University Press, Buckingham, pp. 25–37.

Hermansson, G.L., Webster, A.C. and McFarland, K. (1988) Counselor deliberate postural lean and communication of facilitative conditions. *Journal of Counselling Psychology* **35**, 149–53.

Heron, J. (1989) *Six Category Intervention Analysis*, 3rd ed. (Human Potential Research Project.) University of Surrey, Guildford.

Heron, J. (1990) *Helping the Client – a Creative Practical Guide*. Sage, London.

Honeycutt, J.M. and Worobey, J.L. (1987) Impressions about communication styles and competence in nursing relationships. *Communication Education* **36**, 217–27.

Izard, C.E. (1980) Cross-cultural perspectives on emotion and emotion communication. In *Handbook of Cross-Cultural Psychology: Basic Processes, Vol. 3.* (eds H.C. Triandis and W. Lonner) Allyn and Bacon, Boston, MA.

Jaques, D. (1984) *Learning in Groups*. Croom Helm, London.

Jarvis, P. (1988) *Adult and Continuing Education: Theory and Practice*. Routledge, London.

Kagan, C., Evans, J. and Kay, B. (1986) *A Manual of Interpersonal Skills for Nurses: an Experimental Approach*. Harper & Row, London.

Kiecolt-Glaser, J.K., Glasser, R., Strain, E.C., Strout, J.C., Tarr, K.I., Holliday, J.E. and Speicher, C.E. (1986) Modulation of cellular immunity in medical students. *Journal of Behavioral Medicine* **9**, 5–22.

Knowles, M.S. (1984) Introduction: The art and science of helping adults learn. In *Andragogy in Action*. (ed. M.S. Knowles) Jossey-Bass, San Francisco, pp. 1–21.

Kolb, D. and Fry, R. (1975) Towards an applied theory of experiential learning. In *Theories of Group Processes*. (ed. C.L. Cooper) Wiley, Chichester, pp. 33–56.

Leyens, J-P. and Codol, J-P. (1988) Social cognition. In *Introduction to Social Psychology*. (ed. M. Hewstone, W. Stroebe, J-P. Codol and G.M. Stephenson) Blackwell, Oxford, Chapter 5.

Lovell, R.B. (1982) *Adult Learning*. Croom Helm, London.

Macleod Clark, J. (1981) Patients' needs and nurses' skills. *Nursing* **1**, 1164–65.

Matsumoto, D. (1989) Face, culture, and judgements of anger and fear: do the eyes have it?. *Journal of Nonverbal Behavior*, **13**, 171–88.

Maslow, A.H. (1970) *Motivation and Personality*, 2nd ed. Harper & Row, New York.

McKay, M., Davis, M. and Fanning, P. (1983) *Messages: The Communication Skills Book*. New Harbinger, Oakland, CA.

Mearns, D. and Thorne, B. (1988) *Person Centred Counselling in Action*. Sage, London.

Minardi, H. (1995) *Whether Education has an Effect on the Ability of Health Care Workers to Identify Emotions from Facial Expressions*. (Unpublished BSc Psychology Project) Birkbeck College, University of London, London.

Minardi, H.A. and Riley, M. (1988) Providing psychological safety through skilled communication. *Nursing* **3**, 990–92.

Minardi, H.A. and Riley, M. (1991) The use of team teaching for communication skills training in nurse education. *Nurse Education Today* **11**, 57–64.

Minton, D. (1991) *Teaching Skills in Further and Adult Education*. City and Guilds/ Macmillan, Basingstoke.

Mussen, P.H., Conger, J.J., Kagan, J. and Huston, A.C. (1990) *Child Development and Personality*, 3rd ed. Harper Collins, New York.

Nelson-Jones, R. (1982) *The Theory and Practice of Counselling Psychology*. Cassell, London.

Nursing Standard (1995) News report. *Nursing Standard* 9(43), 10.

Nutbeam, D. (1986) Health promotion glossary. *Health Promotion* 1, 113–27.

Pasquali, E.A., Arnold, H.M. and DeBasio, N. (1989) *Mental Health Nursing: a Holistic Approach*. Mosby, St Louis, MO.

Patton, B.R. and Griffin, K. (1974) *Interpersonal Communication*. Harper & Row, New York.

Pearce, J.M. (1987) *An Introduction to Animal Cognition*. Lawrence Erlbaum, Hove.

Peters, R.S. (1963) *Authority, Responsibility and Education*, 2nd ed. George Allen and Unwin, London.

Peters, R.S. (1966) *Ethics and Education*. George Allen and Unwin, London.

Pfeiffer, J.W. (1985) *Reference Guide to Handbooks and Annuals*. University Associates Publishers and Consultants, San Diego, CA.

Pfeiffer, J.W. and Jones, J.J. (1969–1985) *A Handbook of Structured Experiences for Human Relations Training, Vol. I–X*. University Associates Publishers and Consultants, San Diego, CA.

Philbrick, F.A. (1966) Bias words. In *Introductory Readings on Language*, rev. ed. (eds W.L. Anderson and N.C. Stageberg) Holt, Rinehart and Winston, New York, pp. 176–84.

Porritt, L. (1990) *Interaction Strategies*, 2nd ed. Churchill Livingstone, Melbourne.

Priestly, P., McGuire, J., Flegg, D., Hemsley, V. and Welham, D. (1978) *Social Skills and Personal Problem Solving: a Handbook of Methods*. Tavistock Publications, London.

Quinn, F.M. (1995) *The Principles and Practice of Nurse Education*, 3rd ed. Chapman & Hall, London.

Rachman, S.J. and Philips, C. (1975) *Psychology and Medicine*. Temple Smith, London.

Raymond, D.D., Dowrick, P.W. and Kleinke, C.L. (1993) Affective responses to seeing oneself for the first time on unedited videotape. *Counselling Psychology Quarterly* 6, 193–200.

Rogers, C.R. (1961) *On Becoming a Person – a Therapist's View of Psychotherapy*. Constable, London.

Rogers, C.R. (1980) *A Way of Being*. Houghton Mifflin, Boston, MA.

Rutter, M. (1981) *Maternal Deprivation Reassessed*. Penguin, Harmondsworth.

Saunders, C. (1986) Opening and closing. In *A Handbook of Communication Skills*. (ed. O. Hargie) Routledge, London.

Scheflen, A.E. and Ashcraft, N. (1976) *Human Territories: how we behave in space–time*. Prentice Hall, Englewood Cliffs, NJ.

Schegloff, W. and Sacks, H. (1973) Opening-up closings. *Semiotica* 8, 289–327.

Schön, D.A. (1983) *The Reflective Practitioner: How Professionals Think in Action*. Basic Books, New York.

Slobin, D.I. (1979) *Psycholinguistics*, 2nd ed. Scott, Forseman and Company, Illinois.

Smith, V.L. and Clark, H.H. (1993) On the course of answering questions. *Journal of Memory and Language* **32**, 25–38.

Sternbach, R.A. (1968) *Pain: a Psycho-physiological Analysis*. Academic Press, London.

Sullivan, J.J. (1991) Three roles of language in motivation theory. In *Motivation and Work Behaviour*, 5th ed. (eds R.M. Steers and L.W. Porter) McGraw-Hill, New York, pp. 546–60.

Sundeen, S.J., Stuart, G.W., Rankin, E.A. and Cohen, S.A. (1989) *Nurse–Client Interaction*, 4th ed. Mosby, St Louis, MO.

Sutherland, P. (1992) *Cognitive Development Today: Piaget and His Critics*. Paul Chapman, London.

Townend, A. (1985) *Assertion Training*. FPA Education Unit, London.

Trower, P., Bryant, B. and Argyle, M. (1978) *Social Skills and Mental Health*. Methuen, London.

van Ments, M. (1992) Role-play without tears – some problems of using role-play. *Simulation/Games for Learning* **22**, 82–90.

Vygotsky, L.S. (1962) *Thought and Language*. MIT Press, Cambridge, MA.

Walker, S. (1987) *Animal Learning: an Introduction*. Routledge & Kegan Paul, London.

Watts, F. (1986) Listening to the client. *Changes* (Jan) 164–67.

Weil, S.W. and McGill I., eds. (1989) *Making Sense of Experiential Learning: Diversity in Theory and Practice*. The Society for Research into Higher Education and Open University Press, Buckingham.

Wills, T.A. and Langner, T.S. (1980) Socioeconomic status and stress. In *Handbook of Stress and Anxiety*, (eds I.L. Kutash, C.B. Schlesinger, *et al.*) Jossey-Bass, San Francisco.

Index